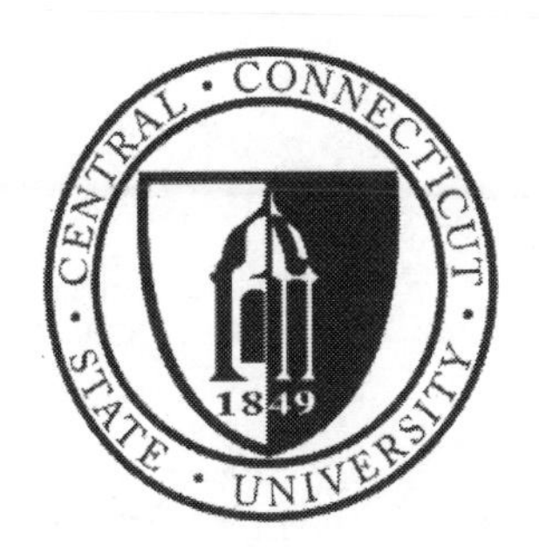

College Wellness

PE 144 – Fitness and Wellness

Editors:

Dr. Cassandra York, R.D.,

Dr. Mike Voight, Professor

Department of Physical Education and Human Performance

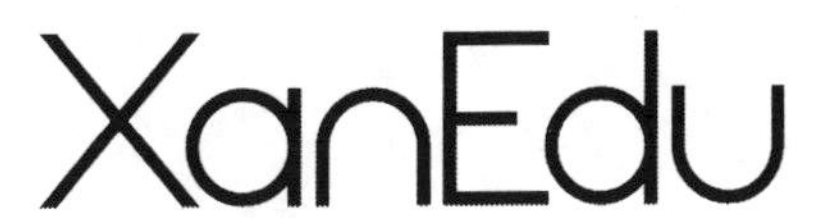

The editors would like to acknowledge Kimberly T. Kostelis, DPE, Interim Dean of the School of Education and Professional Studies at CCSU. This book would not exist without her vision and effort.

Printed in the United States of America

ISBN 13: 978-1-59399-861-5

Acknowledgments:

p. 59: Copyright © University of Kentucky College of Agriculture, Food and Environment.

p. 62: Copyright © 2011, Harvard University. For more information about The Healthy Eating Plate, please see The Nutrition Source, Department of Nutrition, Harvard School of Public Health, www.thenutritionsou ce.org, and Harvard Health Publications, www.health.harvard.edu.

p. 63: As appeared on ThroughTheBurn.com.

p. 98: Copyright © National Alliance on Mental Illness (NAMI). Reprinted by permission.

p. 105: Copyright © Anxiety and Depression Association of America (ADAA). www.adaa.org. Reprinted by permission.

XanEdu
4750 Venture Drive, Suite 400
Ann Arbor, MI 48108
800-562-2147
www.xanedu.com

Table of Contents

Author Bios

Dr. Jan Galen Bishop
An Associate Professor in the Physical Education and Human Performance (PEHP) department with expertise in physical education pedagogy and fitness education. She teaches both undergraduate and graduate courses and is Director of the PEHP Graduate program. She is the author of *Fitness Through Aerobics*, co-author of *Step Up to Wellness*, a Certified Physical Best Instructor, and a National Academy of Sports Medicine (NASM) Certified Personal Trainer.

Mr. Richard Bishop
Is Director of Financial Aid at CCSU. He holds degrees in Finance, Accounting & Management, and worked as a NYSC licensed Stock Broker & Options Trader.

Ms. Carol Ciotto
An Associate Professor in the PEHP department who serves as Program Coordinator for the Physical Education Teacher Education (PETE) Program and as a university supervisor of student teachers. She teaches Elementary Methods of PE and Organization of Curriculum and Program Development at the undergraduate level and teaches Physical Activity and Health Concepts for Physical Educators at the graduate level. Her research interests include brain-based learning through movement, physical activity and the aging, and social and emotional learning.

Dr. Amy G. Gagnon
An Associate Professor in the PEHP department since 2011. Prior to that, she taught physical education for 23 years in the Connecticut public schools. Dr. Gagnon now teaches courses to undergraduates interested in teaching physical education and health as a career. Her areas of expertise are in physical activity for children and how exercise effects learning/social emotional learning environments.

Dr. Tan Leng Goh
An Assistant Professor in the PEHP department. She teaches the lifetime activity, assessment in physical and health education, motor learning and skill acquisition, and methods of teaching school health education courses. Her research focuses on the effects of Comprehensive School Physical Activity Program (CSPAP) on children's physical activity levels, on-task behavior and teachers' perspectives on implementing CSPAP in K-12 schools.

Dr. Jim Malley

An Associate Professor Emeritus and former Chair of the Department of Counselor Education and Family Therapy. He is a founding member of CCSU's Forum for Contemplative Practices and coordinates CCSU's weekly Moment-to-Moment meditation program for CCSU students, faculty, and staff. He teaches a graduate course, Mindfulness in Health & Education, and serves on the School of Education and Professional Studies (SEPS) Advisory Committee for Social and Emotional Learning.

Dr. Matt Martin

An Associate Professor in the PEHP department who teaches undergraduate classes such as Psycho-Social Aspects of PE and Adapted Physical Education. His research interests include examining pedagogical strategies to train Physical Education Teacher Education (PETE) students and inclusive practices for individuals with disabilities.

Mr. Thomas McCarthy

Serves as both Assistant Athletic Trainer for CCSU athletics and an Associate Professor in the PEHP department. He teaches the following undergraduate courses: Care and Treatment of Athletic Injuries, Therapeutic Modalities, Clinical Examination and Diagnosis, and the Practicum in Athletic Training I.

Dr. Jason Melnyk

An Associate Professor in PEHP who teaches graduate classes in Exercise Physiology, and undergraduate courses in Strength and Conditioning, Aging, and Anatomy & Physiology. He is the current President of the New England Chapter of the American College of Sports Medicine (NEACSM) and has a passion for health and fitness. He can be followed on twitter @jmelnyk.

Dr. Pete Morano

An Associate Professor in PEHP who teaches the following undergraduate courses: Introduction to Human Performance, Foundations of Athletic Training, Pharmacology in Sports Medicine, and Fitness/Wellness Ventures. He is the Program Director and Clinical Coordinator for the Athletic Training Education Program.

Dr. Matthew Orange

An Assistant Professor in PEHP teaching Anatomy and Physiology. He is a contributing author to a digital A&P textbook and has published numerous peer-reviewed articles investigating cancer progression and diagnosis and processes governing cell and tissue repair.

Ms. Kathy Pirog

Currently Kathy holds a dual role as the Blue Devil's head Athletic Trainer and Professor of Athletic Training Education in the PEHP department. She has been awarded the University's Distinguished Service Award and a "Women of Influence" award, as well as service awards from the National Athletic Trainers Association (NATA), including membership in the Connecticut Athletic Trainers Associations (CATA) and Eastern Athletic Trainers Associations (EATA) Hall of Fames. She also has held several leadership positions for the CATA.

Dr. Mike Voight

A Professor in the PEHP department who teaches graduate courses in Sport/Exercise Psychology, Leadership, and Sport Sociology, and undergrad courses in Stress Management and Exercise Science. He is the author of 7 books on leadership and mental toughness and consults with top Division I programs on leadership and mental/team toughness. His research areas include leadership and team development. His website is: www.drvleads.com

Dr. Sean Walsh

As a Professor in the PEHP department, he has served in several leadership roles in numerous professional organizations at the state, regional and national levels. He has served as President of the NEACSM and on the Executive Committee of the American College of Sports Medicine (ACSM) Pronouncements Committee. His main area of research has been in Exercise Genomics. Additionally, Dr. Walsh is a Fellow of the ACSM and has received several teaching awards at Central including a four-time Honor Roll for Excellence in Teaching recipient.

Dr. Cassandra York

An Assistant Professor in the PEHP department. She holds her PhD in Kinesiology from UCONN and her MS in Nutrition and Metabolism from the University of Alberta, Canada. She is also a Registered Dietitian (RD) and certified as a Strength and Conditioning Specialist (CSCS) through the NSCA. She has authored three nationally published books: *The New Rules of Lifting for Women,* the *Women's Health Perfect Body Diet*, and the *Prevention No Bloat Diet*. Her research interests are strength training practices for women, and diet for optimal gut health.

Chapter 1

Living Healthy

By Jan Galen Bishop, EdD, Natalie Tamjid, and Sean Walsh, PhD

Chapter Objectives

After reading this chapter, students should be able to:

- ✓ Understand Wellness Dimensions important for college students and life beyond CCSU;
- ✓ Understand the Transtheoretical Model of Behavior Change as it relates to promoting a healthy lifestyle;
- ✓ Understand the benefits of physical activity for a healthy lifestyle;
- ✓ Recognize skills needed to be a successful student at Central Connecticut State University (CCSU).

Living Healthy in College and Beyond

"Take care of your body, it's the only place you'll have to live"- Jim Rohn

Welcome to Central Connecticut State University! We are delighted that you have selected CCSU as your university of choice. College life is full of exploration, change and opportunity. This can be exciting and stressful at times. PE 144 College Wellness is a course designed to assist you in finding a balanced healthy way of living that will optimize your experience in college and prepare you for life beyond.

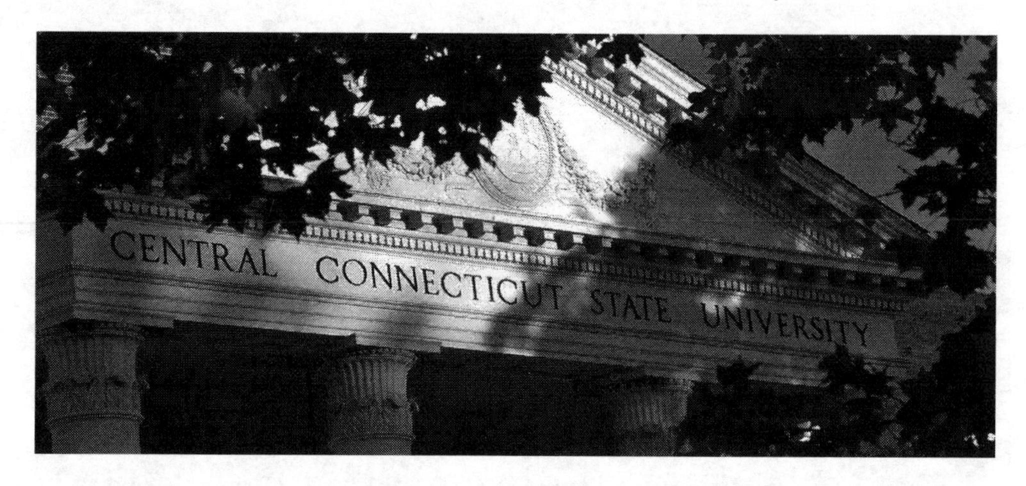

As you explore the many educational career paths available to you, it is important to note that to succeed in any one of them, you will need to develop good habits and make healthy lifestyle choices. Learning to live a wellness lifestyle takes practice and is an ongoing process. Wellness can be defined as a "multidimensional state of being, describing the existence of positive health in an individual as exemplified by quality of life and a sense of wellbeing" (Corbin, Pangrazi, 2001). The eight dimensions of wellness are introduced in this chapter and elaborated on in subsequent chapters. When one dimension is emphasized to the detriment of others, stress mounts. Too often college success is measured by grade point average (intellectual wellness), and while that is certainly important, it is only one aspect of college wellness. Intellectual wellness can only be sustained if the other dimensions such as emotional, social, and physical wellness are also developed and nurtured. The interconnectedness of all the dimensions of wellness is a very important concept.

This course, *PE 144 College Wellness*, is designed to help you identify, develop and strengthen wellness habits, and give you access to the knowledge you will need to make healthy lifestyle decisions. While the goal is to strive for a well-managed and balanced lifestyle, it is equally important to learn how to recover your balance when life's circumstances push you off center. Your instructor and this custom-made textbook will provide you with: 1) up-to-date and relevant wellness information, 2) opportunities to apply and practice what you learn, and 3) campus resources to help you navigate your way through your educational journey here at CCSU.

The Eight Dimensions of Wellness

The eight dimensions of wellness are: physical, spiritual, social, intellectual, environmental, emotional, occupational, and financial (Figure 1).

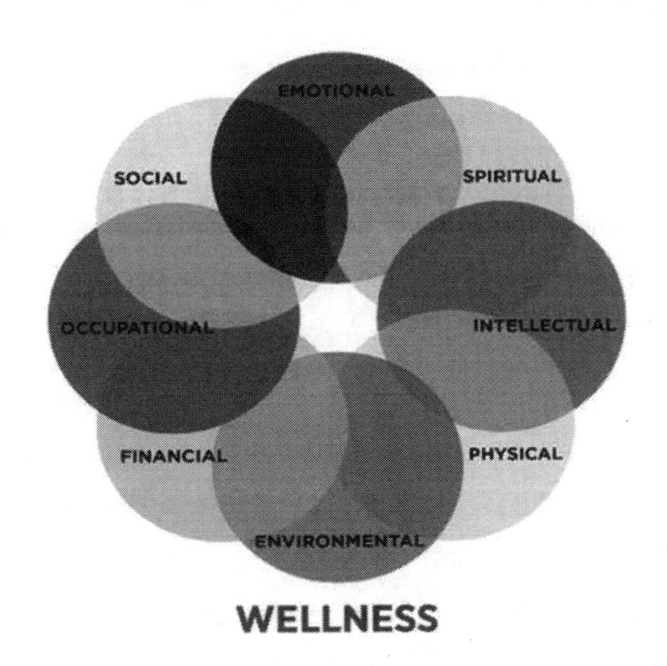

Figure 1. Eight Dimensions of Wellness

Many people tend to place emphasis on a single dimension or just a few dimensions, but as mentioned above, it is important to optimize each aspect of wellness for an overall state of wellbeing. The arrival at a university setting, whether living at the school or commuting, can place several obstacles in the way of your wellness. As a young adult, these challenges can sometimes be overwhelming, but they can be minimized or avoided by focusing on overall wellness. After reading through this section, think about each dimension of wellness and your own individual lifestyle. Identify your strengths and weaknesses and begin to think about what changes you might want to make to become better in one or more of these areas.

Physical Wellness

Physical wellness includes adequate physical activity, proper diet, monitoring alcohol use, and avoiding cigarettes and drugs, in order to obtain and maintain optimal functioning of our body.

Adequate physical activity is lacking in North America, as evidenced by our rapidly increasing rates of overweight and obesity. Inadequate physical activity is closely related to increased morbidity and mortality: individuals with low fitness levels are eight times more likely to die of cardiovascular disease, and five times more likely to die from cancer. However improved health benefits can be achieved even from small increases in activity. An individual who previously took no part in exercise can achieve significant benefits by simply walking for 30 minutes, three times a week.

Health benefits of physical activity include: cardiorespiratory endurance, joint flexibility, muscular strength/endurance, and improved body composition. Additionally, a focus on physical wellness can reduce blood cholesterol, blood pressure, body fat, stress, depression and fatigue; all of which can decrease risk of cardiovascular disease, cancer, diabetes, obesity, and osteoporosis. Regular physical activity can also increase your ability to concentrate and retain information, which is something all students can benefit from. You will learn more about Physical Wellness in Chapter 2.

Nurturing your body by eating a well-balanced diet which provides adequate vitamins and minerals will also help to improve your physical wellness. Aspects of a proper diet include: eating 5½ cups of vegetables and fruits daily, drinking eight 8-oz glasses of water, monitoring portion sizes, focusing on whole grains over processed starches, and only eating 'unhealthy' or 'junk foods' (i.e. cake, cookies, chips) in moderation. Avoiding destructive habits, such as binge-drinking, smoking cigarettes, and taking drugs are also important for physical wellness. Pay attention to your alcohol consumption and understand it is okay to say no when a friend or family member asks you to have a drink. If alcohol is consumed, it should be consumed in moderation (only at legal age), up to one drink per day for women and two drinks per day for men. Avoid tobacco and other drugs at all costs; drugs will have no positive effect on your physical health. Smoking cigarettes is the leading cause of preventable disease, disability and death in the United States. Every year almost half of all Americans will die prematurely due to smoking cigarettes or second-hand smoke exposure.

Spiritual Wellness

When you think of the word "spiritual" what comes to mind? This dimension is not to be confused with referring solely to religion or religious belief. Rather, spiritual wellness refers to developing a sense of purpose and happiness by acquiring a higher quality of life. For some, this may mean identifying your personal weaknesses or opening your mind to new ideas or views. For others, this may mean learning to have empathy towards others, or developing the ability to admit when you are wrong. Whatever the case may be, developing a sense of spiritual wellness is important on your journey to creating a greater quality of life.

Spiritual wellness also includes being able to adapt and respond positively to situations or events that may seem misfortunate. This is important when maintaining a positive outlook on life, for there will be times in life that we are unable to control events that happen. How we view and move forward from these situations is what is important.

Social Wellness

The social dimension of wellness includes interactions between oneself and others. It includes developing nurturing relationships with others and creating loving connections with those around us. Researchers are unsure how love can improve immune function and health; however, multiple studies have concluded that loving relationships do just that. Extended life, improved white blood cells, and improvement in antibodies, among other variables, have all been correlated to experiencing love. When you look at your personal relationships with others, you should focus on the relationships support your social wellness and avoid those that hinder it.

Intellectual Wellness

This dimension of wellness involves the intellectual and creative aspects of our mind. Participating in new experiences and learning new knowledge help to expand and encourage our dimension of intellectual wellness. Welcoming new challenges and engaging in stimulating opportunities will allow your brain to exercise its capacity of thinking. Intellectual wellness also involves the idea of curiosity. Curiosity is healthy and helps to expand our minds, to think clearly, and acquire new knowledge. Being open-minded, listening, and exploring your creativity are all ways to exercise your intellectual wellness.

Environmental Wellness

Environmental wellness requires that individuals live a lifestyle that is respectful to their surrounding environment. This includes being aware of how your daily life is impacting the world around you. Do you recycle? Do you work to conserve energy whenever possible? Do you offer your time to organizations that strive to improve the environment? All the suggestions above can help you improve your environmental wellness.

Emotional Wellness

Your emotional state is made up of the emotions you are feeling at any time. Emotional wellness is the ability to understand, accept, and express how you are feeling to create a positive mind and body.

The mind is a powerful entity that controls many aspects of our quality of life. The mind and the body share a strong relationship and recent research suggests that the mind may play a larger role on the health of our bodies than once thought. For example, when you are feeling stressed and anxious, your body responds with a negative reaction. This reaction may lead to medical complications such as ulcers, high blood pressure, and weight loss/ or gain. On the contrary, focusing on a positive emotional outlook may improve your overall health: Happy mind = Happy body.

Positive self-image is an aspect of emotional wellness that can help you become more confident as a person overall. Improving your self-image, like improving any skill, takes time and practice. Developing good self-esteem involves encouraging a positive (but realistic) attitude toward yourself and the world around you and appreciating your worth, while at the same time behaving responsibly towards others. Self-esteem isn't self-absorption; it's self-respect.

Happiness is one aspect of self-esteem. Happy individuals are capable of loving themselves more often than unhappy individuals. Happiness depends on the individual, and the definition may vary depending on who you talk to. However, most can conclude that being happy contributes to concepts such as positive self-image, self-concept, and confidence. To improve your happiness and overall emotional wellness, communicate your emotional state effectively, take care of yourself, keep a positive mind, remove negative interactions from your life, reflect and relax your mind and body with tools such as meditation, yoga, deep breathing, and regular daily exercise. Chapter 5 will give you a greater view of emotional wellness

Occupational Wellness

This dimension of wellness involves finding fulfillment in your career path and balancing your job or school life with your leisure time. Finding a career that is consistent with your goals and desires is important when establishing your occupational wellness. Your career will be rewarding when it is in line with your passions and when you ensure to include enjoyable time away from work; take time to let yourself to unwind and destress after work by leaving time for socializing, spending time with your family, and your enjoying your hobbies or other free time activities.

Financial Wellness

This dimension of wellness addresses being financially secure, in both your present and future life. Financial stability is achieved by being able to budget and by monitoring and tracking spending and saving. Developing an understanding between "needs" and "wants" can help distinguish between necessary and unnecessary costs in your daily life. Achieving financial wellness can help create a sense of comfort and can help lower stress related to money. This dimension of wellness also includes having awareness and knowledgeable of all financial options, such as opening a savings account, acquiring loans or a credit card, and options for school financial aid including scholarships, grants, and loans. Chapter 8 goes into detail about Financial Wellness.

Transtheoretical Model of Behavior Change

As you read through the dimensions of wellness, you may have identified an area you would like to improve. This will mean breaking old habits and building new ones. For many, changing one's behavior, especially if it is ingrained, is not easy, but that does not mean changing a behavior is impossible. Researchers have dug into what helps people change and the result has been a number of theories and practices, one of which is the *Transtheoretical Model of Behavior Change*. This is the one we will use in this course. It can be very helpful and applied to several different behaviors.

You may be thinking, "Why should I bother changing my unhealthy behaviors? I feel I am doing OK". While this may be true, altering your lifestyle to adopt healthy behaviors will allow you to improve your quality of life even more. In other words, a healthy lifestyle will help decrease your risk of disease, expand the length of your life, and improve your overall health, happiness and wellness.

As mentioned, making lifestyle changes is not always easy. However, success can be obtained by gradually progressing through the five stages of the Transtheoretical Model. For some behaviors you may need to start at stage one, for others you may be further along. The five stages include (see Figure 2):

1) Precontemplation
2) Contemplation
3) Preparation
4) Action
5) Maintenance

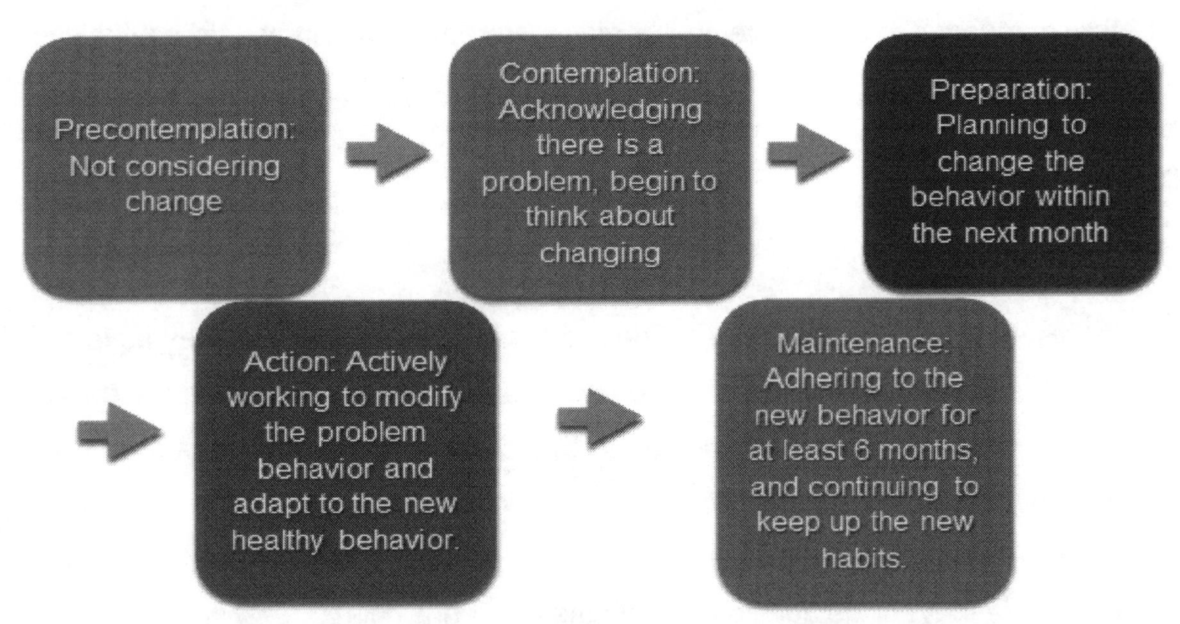

Figure 2. The 5 stages of the Transtheoretical Model of Change

We are going to move through each stage of change, using physical activity as the example in this setting, however, remember that this model can be applied to any health and wellness behavior adaptation.

Precontemplation

In this stage, individuals have no intention of changing their behavior. They often do not understand that their current behavior is unhealthy, harmful, risky, or simply, they do not care. Most individuals in this stage stick to the idea that the cons of changing outweigh the benefits. For example, people in this stage feel that taking time out of their day to exercise is not worth the health benefits because they would lose precious time that they could spend doing anything else other than exercise.

Contemplation

Individuals in this stage often are unsure of whether or not they wish to change their behavior. They are considering the benefits of changing yet have not committed to making the change. They often find the pros and cons of changing equal and are not fully persuaded to either side. In this stage, individuals would be unsure if taking time to exercise is worth what will result.

Preparation

In this stage, individuals have decided to change their behavior. They have decided that the pros outweigh the cons and intend to initiate the changes in the near future (30 days or less). Often individuals in this stage have started to take small steps toward their goals but have not begun their full plan of action yet. In this stage, individuals will begin to see that taking time to exercise is worth it. However, they may be unsure they will be able to maintain the new behavior.

Action

In this stage, individuals have recently changed their behavior in the last six months and intend to continue to adapt to the healthy behavior. They have a plan and are consistent with this new behavior. However, individuals in this stage are at risk of relapse. Relapse is when an individual reverts back to their previous unhealthy behavior. Individuals in this stage clearly see that the benefits of exercise have completely outweighed any cons.

Maintenance

In this stage, individuals have maintained their new behavior for longer than six months. They have recognized the benefits that have come from the change and have made the change a part of their lifestyle. They are less likely to experience relapse and have fewer temptations to revert to their previous habits. They are confident with their new behavior and intend to continue the behavior moving forward.

Moving from Stage to Stage

PRECONTEMPLATION → CONTEMPLATION

Precontemplators often are unaware of the benefits of adapting to the new behavior. For example, the benefits of engaging in physical activity would result in improved fitness, decreased body fat, increased body satisfaction, body image, self-concept, as well as reduced risk of several diseases, such as cardiovascular disease, diabetes, some cancers. Educating precontemplators on the many benefits that would come with a behavior change may help to persuade change. In some cases, precontemplators may be aware of these benefits, but the barriers to overcome the change may seem too time consuming, too difficult, or unnecessary.

Barriers are the challenges that precontemplators are often trying to avoid. Such as: 'none of my friends' exercise', or 'I have no energy left by the end of the day to exercise.' To combat these barriers, supports are needed. Supports are the positive result from overcoming barriers making it worth the challenge. Supports can be anything from improved health, improved self-esteem, monetary rewards, or improved self-efficacy (the belief that you are capable of completion).

Activity #1: Barriers to Exercise

List out potential barriers to engaging in physical activity.

A sample is provided below.

1) *Too tired to exercise*
2)
3)
4)
5)

List out potential ways you can overcome these barriers.

A sample is provided below.

1) *Schedule exercise at the time of day when you are most energized. For some, this may mean exercising in morning time before heading to work, for others this may mean exercising at nighttime after dinner. Find what works best for you and move forward from there.*
2)
3)
4)
5)

CONTEMPLATION → PREPARATION

To motivate contemplators to make a change in their physical activity habits they may benefit from: Increased awareness of the benefits of physical activity, support from friends and peers, and identifying specific goals for the future. Goals should be broken down into small and manageable behaviors. For example, instead of making a goal 'to be physically fit', a better goal would be 'to walk the dog three days a week for 30 minutes' or 'to attend a cardio dance class twice a week with a friend'. By breaking goals into smaller more manageable steps, you will be able to monitor and track your successes and avoid feeling overwhelmed.

PREPARATION → ACTION

To move from preparation to action you will need to make a plan. Referencing back to the concept of barriers, barriers identified must be addressed and a plan must be set to overcome each of them. With a plan in place, you will be more successful. Example: If your barrier was time, take one day and write down everything you did in a journal. Evaluate and analyze how you are spending your time. Most likely there are things that can be eliminated. For example, did you sit on your bed and aimlessly switch back and forth through social media platforms? Twitter to Instagram, to Kik, back to Instagram...and so on and so forth. How much time was spent doing this? Keep in mind dedicating time to improve health can take as little as 30 minutes a day.

ACTION → MAINTENANCE

To move from the action stage to the maintenance stage you must adhere to the new healthy behavior for at least six months. After six months, the behavior should become habit, and likely will be implemented into your permanent lifestyle. The maintenance stage requires consistent motivation and commitment to continue on your new health path.

Facilitating a Behavior Change

Listed below are a few ways to help support you on your path to changing unhealthy behaviors.

CONSCIOUS-RAISING: The first step in modifying a behavior is to understand why the problem behavior is bad for you. Learning why adapting the new behavior will benefit you will increase your likelihood of adherence.

- ✓ The current course will provide you with the knowledge to understand the importance of health and wellness.
- ✓ Visit the Health and Wellness Center on campus

COUNTERING: Process of substituting a healthy behavior for a problem behavior.

- ✓ Drinking water instead of soda.
- ✓ Eat carrots instead of potato chips.
- ✓ Walking instead of driving.
- ✓ Playing billiards at the student center instead of watching TV and snacking.
- ✓ Dancing or moving instead of sitting while talking on the phone.

SOCIAL LIBERATION: The act of gaining social support for positive change.

- ✓ Joining a group fitness class offered by RECentral.
- ✓ Using exercise facilities that are open during recreation times.
- ✓ Linking up with others and creating a "fitness club" or "workout group"
- ✓ Placing healthy foods/drinks in your car, backpack, or home.
- ✓ Eating out at places that have choices that include healthy foods.
- ✓ Buying the clothing needed to be active comfortably outside in all weather.

ENVIORNMENTAL CONTROL: The process of reducing temptations and controlling the environment to promote healthy choices.

- ✓ Throw away all junk food in the house.
- ✓ Purchase plenty of vegetables and fruits each time you grocery shop

- ✓ Staying away from friends who use drugs
- ✓ Perform exercises that can be done anywhere. For example:
    - Wall sits while waiting between classes
    - Push-ups with feet (or hands) on a sturdy piece of furniture
    - Squats and lunges while waiting for food to cook
    - Jumping jacks or jogging in place while watching TV
- ✓ Using the warm water of a shower/tub/sauna to prepare you for stretching.
- ✓ Linking flexibility exercises to times when you have been active. For example, after walking across campus:
    - Take a minute to stretch calves or hamstrings.
        - Place foot up on a stair and lean forward.
        - Stand on a stair on balls of feet; drop heels down.
    - Stop in doorways; grab with your hands to stretch shoulders/chest.

HELPING RELATIONSHIPS: The process of surrounding yourself with people who will support you move toward your goals.

- ✓ Commit to exercising with a friend or group of friends.
- ✓ Carpool to the gym. When it is your turn to drive, it's harder not to show up!
- ✓ Eating out with friends who make healthy, nutritious choices
- ✓ Spending time with people who improve your happiness instead of bringing you down

Activity #2: Behavior Change

Chose a behavior that you wish to change and answer the following questions.

1) I aim to change the following behavior:________________________
    i. Explain specifically how you want to change (i.e. I would like to exercise for 3 days a week for 30 minutes each day)

2) I chose to change this behavior because:________________________

3) Have you previously tried to change this behavior? If yes, explain what you did and why it did not work? ____________________

4) If I successfully changed this behavior what benefits will I gain?
   a. ____________________
   b. ____________________
   c. ____________________
5) If I fail to change this behavior what consequences will there be?
   a. ____________________
   b. ____________________
   c. ____________________
6) Some *barriers* I may encounter as I work toward my goals may be?
   a. ____________________
   b. ____________________
   c. ____________________
7) Some *supports* I may encounter as I work toward my goals may be?
   a. ____________________
   b. ____________________
   c. ____________________
8) Explain your plan of action? ____________________
   i. Explain specifically how you are going to work toward accomplishing your goal? (i.e. *I will keep a journal to monitor my exercise. I will wake up early to leave time for the gym three days a week*)

Setting Yourself Up for Success

An important first step on your university journey is being able to picture your future. That picture may change along the way as it is common for students to change majors and career goals.

The next step is learning how to set goals, and then use those goals to create a series of steps that will move you toward that picture you have of your future self. It is important to acknowledge that success does not come easily; it isn't handed out; it is earned. The good news is that you are not on this journey alone – faculty, staff, and other students can all play supporting roles. It is important, however, to take personal responsibility for your future. Once you have successfully attained this skill, all other skills should come easier. Begin by meeting with an advisor or mentor within your departmental study of choice. Share with them your goals, why you are here, and why you feel that CCSU is the institution that will allow you to successfully accomplish the future you are picturing. In each of your courses this semester, review the course syllabus and take note of important dates and percentage points of each assignment or test. Be ready to attend and take notes in all your classes. But most importantly, surround yourself with likeminded individuals who will help you reach your goals and PLAN for success. Share this plan with family, friends, and faculty while seeking out advice along the way. Build yourself an educational network of these individuals who will help you achieve the academic goals that you are putting forth! These are all items that will become important as you become an independent learner here at CCSU.

In addition, be sure to take time to build friendships. Social and emotional health comes from feeling connected and supported. CCSU offers many club and recreational activities that are free for students.

To assess your current actions that will set you up for success, go through the activity below. After completing it, reflect on which items need improvement and how you can change them.

Activity #3: Personal Success Evaluation

The following is a list of actions which are important for success here at CCSU.

- Write a + next to the items you feel you can do well.
- Write a 0 next to the items you feel you need more help with.

___ Envision your future and be able to articulate it

___ Prepare for that future by identify steps to take to get there

___ Work hard – study 3 hours for every hour of lecture

___ Take personal responsibility for your future

___ Go to class – good attendance is a predictor of academic success

___ Read the syllabus for each class and create a calendar for assignments

___ Use a planner

___ Take notes in class

___ Prepare for exams over time (as opposed to cramming the night before)

___ Form study groups

___ Go to professors' office hours

___ Develop a relationship with a mentor in your major

___ Be physically active every day.

___ Eat nutritious meals on a regular basis.

___ Find and use campus services as needed such as the Learning Center, Writing Center, Counseling and Wellness Center

Reflect on who can assist you in improving the areas you marked with a "0":

Health and Wellness Tips

1. **Eat well!** Learning how to cook independently, or at least choose food wisely, is one of the best things that college students can do to improve their health and well-being. Along with this, it is very important to keep in mind what would be good and healthy snacks to eat that will help you get through the day to day activities of college life. Chapter 3 will help you understand good choices.

2. **Exercise!** Physical activity is critical for both a healthy body and mind. The most important thing to realize here is to get involved with activities that you enjoy the most as this can impact your adherence to such an activity.

3. **Study breaks!** Firstly, you need to study to have a break from studying! But if you plan accordingly, hopefully can incorporate small study breaks into your preparations for this can significantly impact your mental health!

4. **Healthy social life!** Social life can be a large aspect of a college community. It is important that you try and develop this aspect of your life. Whether it be forming study groups, joining a club, or getting involved in your community the best way you see fit. These are all aspects that can lead to living a healthier social life.

5. **Limiting alcohol (if over 21) and avoiding drugs!** It is important to surround yourself with individuals who have similar values as you. You are often influenced by the company that you keep. Choose your friends wisely and consider the effects of their friendship on your choices.

Chapter Summary

- ✓ Wellness is multidimensional, and it is important to develop and balance the eight dimensions to have optimize your health, maintain a high quality of life, and enjoy a sense of wellbeing.
- ✓ There are 8 dimensions of wellness that all contribute to a healthy overall lifestyle. They include physical, spiritual, social, intellectual, emotional, environmental, financial and occupational wellness.
- ✓ The five stages of the Transtheoretical Model of Behavior Change are:
    - Precontemplation;
    - Contemplation;
    - Preparation;
    - Action; and
    - Maintenance.
- ✓ Some strategies to help support you with your behavior change are social liberation, conscious raising, countering, environmental control, and helping relationships.
- ✓ To become a successful student at CCSU consider the following suggestions:
    - Take responsibility for your future;
    - Meet with your advisor;
    - Take notes and attend all classes, review each syllabus and make note of important dates and information; and
    - Surround yourself with positive likeminded individuals.

Chapter Review Questions

1) Describe a person who would be in the 'precontemplation' stage.
2) Describe a person who would be in the 'action' stage.
3) List three suggestions that could help you become successful at CCSU.
4) What are barriers? What are supports?

5) What are the minimum recommendations for moderate and vigorous intensity exercise as put forth by the American College of Sports Medicine?
6) Why is it important to understand the 8 dimensions of wellness? After reading about each dimension, is there one that stuck out to you most? In other words, is there one or two dimensions that you feel you need to work on more than others?
7) Choose 2 of the 8 dimensions and describe them. List some ways you can improve your wellness in these dimensions.

References

Alcohol and Public Health. (2017, July 25). Retrieved from **https://www.cdc.gov/alcohol/fact-sheets/moderate-drinking.htm**

Bishop, J. G., & Aldana, S. G. (1999). *Step up to wellness: A stage-based approach.* Boston, MA: Allyn and Bacon.

Corbin, C.B. & Pangrazi, R.P. (2001, December). Toward a Uniform Definition of Wellness: A Commentary. *President's Council on Physical Fitness and Sports Research Digest*. Series 3, n15.

Environmental Wellness. (n.d.). Retrieved from **https://shcs.ucdavis.edu/wellness/environmental**

Environmental Wellness. (n.d.). Retrieved from **https://wellness.ucr.edu/environmental_wellness.html**

Smoking & Tobacco Use. (2017, September 05). Retrieved from **https://www.cdc.gov/tobacco/data_statistics/index.htm**

Social Wellness. (n.d.). Retrieved from **https://shcs.ucdavis.edu/wellness/social**

Physical Wellness. (n.d.). Retrieved from **https://shcs.ucdavis.edu/wellness/physical**

US Department of Health and Human Services (2018). *Physical activity guidelines for Americans, 2015-2018.* **http://www.health.gov/PAGuidelines**.

Chapter 2

Physical Wellness

By Jan Galen Bishop, EdD and Jason Melnyk, PhD

Chapter Objectives

After reading this chapter, students should be able to:

- ✓ Identify the benefits of physical activity;
- ✓ Identify the 4 health-related and 6 skill-related components of fitness and provide examples of each health-related component;
- ✓ Understand the 6 principles of exercise;
- ✓ Apply the recommended exercise guidelines to their own daily physical activity routine
- ✓ Select and use at least one method of tracking intensity in both cardiovascular and resistance training exercise;
- ✓ Understand the movement pattern category of resistance training;
- ✓ Explain the relationship between mobility and stability; and
- ✓ Know where and how to exercise on CCSU's campus.

Physical Wellness

"When it comes to eating right and exercising, there is no 'I'll start tomorrow.' Tomorrow is disease" - V.L Allinear

As we learned in Chapter 1, physical wellness relates to the optimal functioning of our body. This involves all systems including our cardiovascular (heart and lungs), respiratory, digestive, endocrine, muscular and skeletal systems, and how these systems respond to physical activity, diet, and other outside influences.

Regular activity and exercise are a vital part of maintaining a healthy body along with good nutrition and managing physical risk by doing smart things like, limiting alcohol consumption, using suntan lotion, driving responsibly, and practicing safe sex. Physical activity alone has the added benefit of impacting several other wellness dimensions such as:

- **Social & Emotional Wellness:** Physical activities can lift your mood, reduce depression, and provide a healthy environment in which to meet other people.
- **Financial & Occupational Wellness:** Physical activity has been shown to reduce workplace absenteeism and lower health care costs.
- **Spiritual Wellness:** Regular physical activity helps you respond to and better adapt to stressful or misfortunate situations.
- **Intellectual Wellness:** Interspersing physical activity with studying has been shown to improve concentration and retention of information.

It is important to note that physical wellness is something that everyone, including those suffering from disease, can strive for. For example, some people have been successful alleviating chronic pain through yoga and meditation. Physical activity also has a very positive role in weight control and circulation for those with diabetes. Good nutrition can be followed by any person and can help maintain a healthy weight and ward off disease. Avoiding drugs and monitoring alcohol use are also beneficial choices for the health of your body.

Benefits of Physical Activity

According to the Centers for Disease Control and Prevention (2009), regular physical activity can help:

- ✓ Control your weight
- ✓ Reduce your risk of cardiovascular disease
- ✓ Reduce your risk for type 2 diabetes and metabolic syndrome
- ✓ Reduce your risk of some cancers
- ✓ Strengthen your bones and muscles
- ✓ Improve your mental health and mood
- ✓ Improve ability to do daily activities and prevent falls, if you're an older adult
- ✓ Increase your chances of living longer

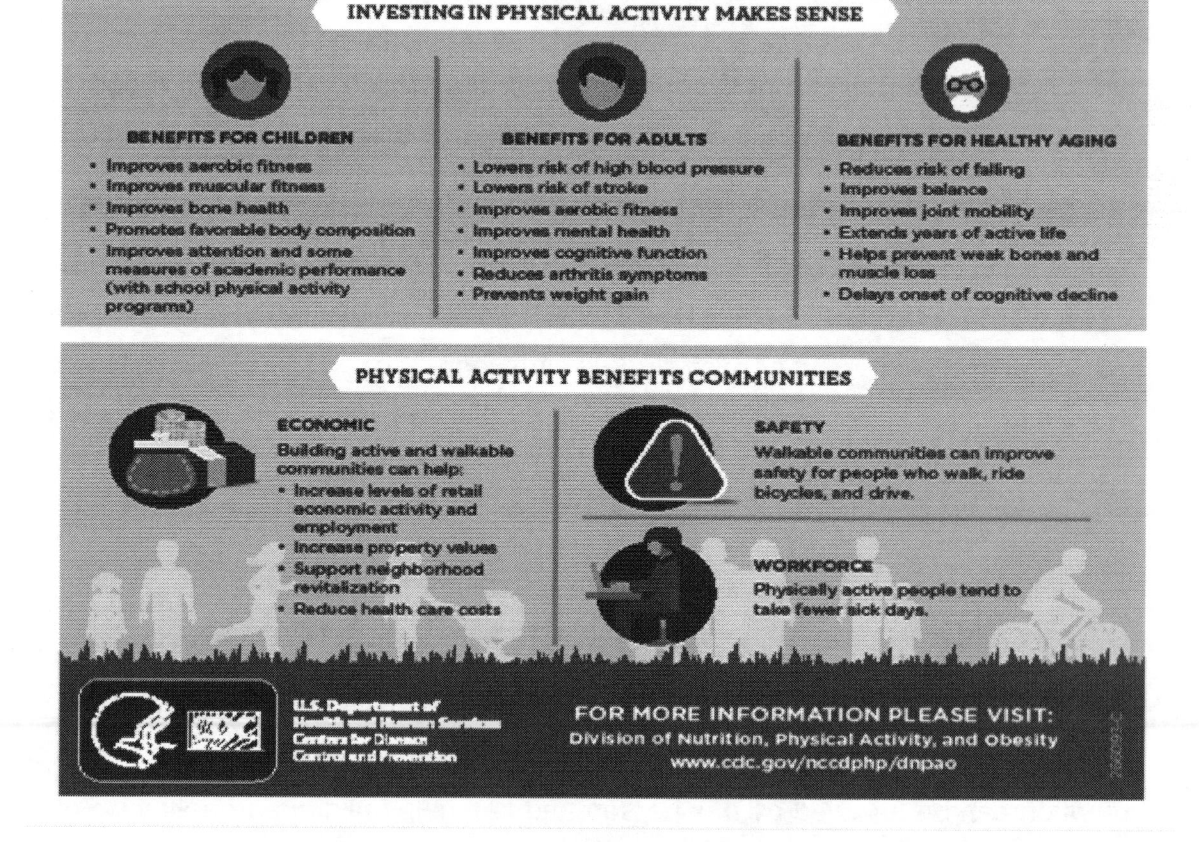

Figure 1. Benefits of Physical Activity

If you're not sure about becoming active or boosting your level of physical activity because you're afraid of getting hurt, the good news is that moderate-intensity aerobic activity, like brisk walking, is generally safe for most people. If you're new to physical activity, start slowly and gradually increase your level of activity over time. If you try to jump into intense exercise too quickly, you may be so sore the next day that you won't want to move. This soreness will go away, so don't let it stop you from continuing after you have healed.

Each of you comes to this class with your own background in physical activity, some of you may be well-versed in exercise and may be a student-athlete here at CCSU; or played a sport or two while in high school; or you may have excelled in your physical education courses in elementary, middle, or high school. Others of you might be more tentative of physical activity and sports. Regardless of your background, the goal is to incorporate enjoyable physical activity into your daily routine so that you can reap the many benefits of a physically active lifestyle. If you do this, in addition to a toned and healthy body, you will have more energy, will be able to concentrate better, and experience less stress.

If you have a chronic health condition, such as arthritis, diabetes, or heart disease, talk with your doctor to find out if your condition limits, in any way, your ability to be active. Then, work with your doctor to come up with a physical activity plan that matches your abilities. If your condition stops you from meeting the minimum guidelines, try to do as much as you can. What's important is that you avoid being inactive. Even 60 minutes a week of moderate-intensity aerobic activity is good for you. That is just 10 minutes a day, 6 days a week. The bottom line is, the health benefits of physical activity far outweigh any potential risks.

Health & Skill-Related Components of Fitness

Many people have a singular idea of what fitness (in relation to physical activity), means. It is often associated with doing bodyweight or aerobic exercises like push-ups or jumping jacks. In fact, fitness is made up of 4 health-related and 6 skill-related components that can be achieved through a combination of activities such as yoga, rock climbing, hiking, swimming, weight-training and all kinds of group fitness activities like cardio-kickboxing, Zumba™, and spinning (cycling). Once you understand the components of fitness and decide what you want to achieve, then you can select activities that appeal to you to accomplish your fitness goals.

Before explaining the components, it is important to understand the differences and similarities between the terms "physical activity", "exercise" and "fitness". Physical activity (PA) is the broadest term and includes any movement that activates your muscles and requires energy. Exercise is a subcategory of PA and is generally thought of as a planned program with set goals to improve health or skill components of fitness. Fitness is a state of being, the more fit you are, the more you can do without getting tired and the better you are able to live free from chronic diseases and illness. It is helpful to focus on the dynamic process of gaining and maintaining fitness and to know how to restart if you have stopped. Events in life such as an illness, accident or feast-laden holiday can temporarily interfere with your fitness plans and even cause you to lose fitness. But as long as the "process" of fitness, including goal-setting, is part of your lifestyle, you can jump back in, and keep the process working for you. As you travel through life, your fitness goals may also change. You may have been a competitive athlete or performance dancer in high school and now may be more interested in just staying active, and not putting on the "freshman 15 pounds".

In 2018, guidelines were published for healthy Americans by the Office of Disease Prevention and Health Promotion that encourage adults to either be moderately active for 150 minutes a week or vigorously active for 75 minutes a week. These guidelines go on to say that combinations of moderate and vigorous intensity exercise can be performed to meet these recommendations and that moderate intensity of activity can be accumulated in as little as three 10-minute bouts of activity throughout the day. The frequency, intensity, and length of time you do activities will determine the fitness level you achieve. Exercise guidelines are discussed in more detail a little later in this chapter.

As stated, the components of fitness are divided into two categories: health-related and skill-related. The former is what this chapter will focus on the most as many people are interested in achieving enough fitness to be healthy. However, skill-components should not be undervalued as they are very important to success in a lot of recreational activities and competitive sports. In addition, the skill-related components of balance and coordination are important in all kinds of functional movements. Being able to catch your balance can also prevent injury. In this text, the health-related components will be numbered as four, however, in some readings you will find them listed as five (this occurs when muscular fitness is identified as two separate components: muscular strength, and muscular endurance).

The HEALTH-RELATED COMPONENTS are:

1) Cardiorespiratory Fitness;
2) Muscular Fitness (strength and endurance);
3) Flexibility; and
4) Body Composition.

The SKILL-RELATED COMPONENTS are:

1) Agility;
2) Balance;
3) Coordination;
4) Power;
5) Reaction Time; and
6) Speed.

To help clarify the difference between health- and skill-related components, here are a couple of examples:

- ✓ Health-related benefits: being able to cycle for 20 minutes without stopping develops your circulatory and respiratory systems (cardiorespiratory fitness), burns calories, provides an energy lift and mentally refreshes you. Cycling will also help develop your leg muscles (muscular fitness/endurance).
- ✓ Skill-related benefits. Being able to go fast (speed) and change directions very quickly (agility) will help you be a competitive and skilled soccer player or hip-hop dancer.

We can assess the optimal functioning of our body by performing tests or assessments of health and skill-related components of fitness. For example, if we performed a 12-minute Cooper test, the objective would be to walk, jog, and/or run the greatest distance possible in the time allowed. An optimal or above average distance covered for a college freshman aged 18 would be to complete approximately 1.8 miles for men or 1.3 miles for women in 12 minutes (Cooper 1968). Ideally you will want to do your own assessments and set goals to improve or maintain your fitness.

Although participating in both recreational and competitive skill-related activities will result in health benefits; the takeaway point is that you don't have to be highly skilled to be healthy. One reason Zumba™, became a popular health-fitness trend was because it deemphasized the "correctness" or skillfulness of steps in favor of energetic movement. This allowed people to become less self-conscious and enjoy the activity.

Cardiorespiratory Fitness

This component is often referred by several names including: cardiorespiratory endurance, cardiovascular fitness (or just cardio for short). It may also be referred to as aerobic fitness, which is one form of cardiorespiratory training; the other major form being anaerobic exercise. Aerobic exercise is continuous rhythmic large muscle activity performed over a prolonged length of time, such as distance running, swimming, and brisk walking. Anaerobic exercise is higher in intensity, so it is performed in short fast bursts of energy. Aerobic exercise is a little gentler as it is done at a lower intensity, which many people enjoy, but recently interval training techniques like HIIT (high intensity interval training) and Tabata have become popular trends especially among young adults.

Muscular Fitness

This component is sometimes referred to as two separate health-related components: *muscular strength* and *muscular endurance*. Muscular strength is the ability to exert maximal effort one time, or near maximal effort over a brief amount of time. An example of this would be one big push to a car stuck in mud or snow or lifting a heavy couch to get the rug under. Muscular endurance is being able to repeat a movement several times (i.e. two-minute push-up test) or hold a position for an extended amount of time (i.e. one-two minute plank hold). These two types of muscular endurance are used in a lot of daily activities, such as carrying grocery bags (holding a weight with arms in one position for an extended time) while walking up 3 flights of stairs (repetitive leg motion). While muscular fitness can be achieved through daily activity, this often results in muscle imbalances (stronger dominant arm, chest stronger than back etc.) so it is important to do things to balance your musculature. For example, after sitting at the computer for a while, purposely pull your shoulder blades together and hold for 6 seconds, relax and repeat 5-10 times. This will counterbalance the forward shoulder position and help develop upper back muscles.

One way to picture the relationship between muscular strength and endurance is to think of a continuum with maximal strength on one end and muscular endurance on the other.

Health-Related Muscular Fitness

↓

Strength ←——————————→ **Muscular Endurance**

To build strength you must move a heavy resistance a few times (1-6 times) while to build muscular endurance you need to move (or hold) a low to moderate resistance a higher number of times (15-25+). In other words, strength requires high load and low repetitions, while endurance requires low-moderate load and high repetitions. As you will learn later in this chapter, health-related guidelines fall in the middle so that you are obtaining a combination of strength and endurance.

Another term associated with muscular fitness is power. Power is the combination of strength and speed. Fast explosive motions like kicking a ball hard or jumping high require power. Note that power is a skill-related component, rather than a health-related one. You don't usually need power to be healthy, but it is very useful in sports and activities like sprinting up the stairs or chopping wood.

Specific resistance training programs are an excellent way to build and maintain muscular fitness. The resistance can come from a variety of sources, such as body weight, dumbbells, medicine balls, kettlebells, barbells, weight training machines, water, etc. Exercises can be carried out in a special gym or right in your dorm/apartment room. It is important to find a way to achieve muscular fitness that appeals to you. One student will be in heaven with a barbell in hand, while another will prefer water aerobics or Pilates™.

Flexibility

Flexibility is defined as the range of motion (ROM) one has around a joint. Take for example the shoulder joint; people with good flexibility can move their arms all the way up overhead, behind them, and out to the side in nice full motions without any pain. If we become sedentary, our muscles begin to lose their elasticity and ROM decreases. This can result in moving poorly, using compensating movements, and may ultimately lead to injury. While there is some loss of elasticity of muscles and tendons with aging, most of the loss is due to lack of movement. Therefore, it is important to stretch and bend most days of the week and do so with both sides of the body: move right and left, forward and backward, and in axial patterns (turning to the right and left). Being able to move freely allows you to do skilled movements correctly, functional movements more easily, and helps prevent both chronic (long-lasting) and acute (short-term) pain and injury. Flexibility is also referred to as mobility. Developing mobility and stability are discussed later in the chapter.

Body Composition

The human body is composed of lean body mass (LBM) and fat mass (FM). Lean body mass includes things like bones, muscle, organs and connective tissue. Fat is found throughout the body and in the right amounts is critical to health. It provides insulation and protection and is a good source of fuel for energy production. Body composition refers to the percentage of LBM and FM.

There are two ways to change body composition: nutrition and physical activity. Good nutrition can reduce fat and support the building of muscles. Physical activity can assist in calorie burning resulting in weight loss or it can build muscle which increases lean body mass. Both will result in a better body composition.

It should be noted that too little fat can be dangerous. Body builders cut their fat levels very low right before competition to highlight muscle definitions. They must be very careful doing this and it is not healthy to stay that lean for any length of time. As with most things, a good balance is the answer. The percentage of body fat can be estimated using skinfold measures, or a Bod Pod, or using an electrical impedance device to check if you are at a healthy level. See Chapter 3 for more information.

Activity #1: Attaining Health-Related Fitness

List 2-3 activities you could do to meet each of the following:

CARDIORESPIRATORY FITNESS

1. ______________________
2. ______________________
3. ______________________

MUSCULAR FITNESS

1. ______________________
2. ______________________
3. ______________________

FLEXIBILITY

1. ______________________
2. ______________________
3. ______________________

BODY COMPOSITION

1. ______________________
2. ______________________
3. ______________________

Principles of Exercise

There are some very useful “rules” to follow when designing or following an exercise plan. These rules are referred to as principles of exercise and when used correctly they will optimize your fitness efforts. Each of the principles is described below along with examples of how they apply to the health-related components of fitness.

PRINCIPLE OF INDIVIDUALITY: This principle embodies the idea that no two people are alike and that they will respond differently to exercise. For example, how one person's body responds to physical activity in terms of weight loss or strength gains can vary widely. Similarly, some people must work much harder than others to develop flexibility. It is important to realize everyone will respond differently even if the same physical activity program is performed. Knowing this, try not to compare yourself to others; rather focus on the gains that you are making and adjust your exercise program to fit you.

PRINCIPLE OF SPECIFICITY: When an activity is performed, it will result in a particular (specific) adaptation by the body. For example, doing push-ups results in muscular strength/endurance to the chest and arms; push-ups do not improve leg strength or increase aerobic capacity. Matching the right exercises to your fitness goals will result in the gains you want. Another term for this is the SAID Principle which stands for Specific Adaptation for Imposed Demand. In other words, pick the exercises (imposed demands) that will result in your desired outcome (specific adaptations).

PRINCIPLE OF OVERLOAD: If improvement is the goal, an exercise must be a little harder than before. It is possible to make exercise harder in a variety of ways, such as doing more of something, or making it more intense, or going longer. Examples would be to do more push-ups, and/or make the push-ups harder by putting the feet up on a bleacher, or by holding the down position of each push-up for 3 seconds before coming up. Aerobic examples would be increasing a run from 1 to 1.5 miles, or running on an incline, or increasing from 15 minutes of running to 20 minutes. Overload can be changing just one aspect or through a combination of aspects.

PRINCIPLE OF PROGRESSION: This principle is generally combined with the Principle of Overload and referred to as the Principle of Progressive Overload. In essence, progression means to do something over time. It is important to exercise consistently over time, but in addition to that if you wish to improve you will want to gradually overload over time. As an example, 10 push-ups can be performed on the knees the first week. On week two, either 12-15 push-ups can be done or perhaps 2 on the toes and the rest of the 10 on the knees. Overtime, the number on the toes can be increased. Too often people try to overload too much or too quickly. This can lead to a lot of soreness or even injury. Applying this principle to aerobic exercise could mean starting with brisk walking for a half a mile, increasing to a whole mile, then alternating jogging and brisk walking to build up to jogging the whole mile.

PRINCIPLE OF REGULARITY: This principle is summed up by the phrase, "Use it or lose it." The benefits of exercise only stick around if you stick to being active. Keeping exercise/physical activity a regular part of your life is central to being healthy.

THE FITT PRINCIPLE: After you decide what you like to do, you will need to use this principle to decide how often, how intensely, and how long to do it. The letters stand for: Frequency, Intensity, Time, and Type. Recently volume and progression have been added to this one making it FITT-VP. Volume is the product of frequency, intensity, and time. Progression means increasing any one of the FITT components. The guidelines section later in the chapter will discuss how to vary the FITT components to align with your starting fitness level and progress to your goal.

Physical Activity Guidelines

As mentioned, engaging in physical activity has many benefits to one's health. It is important to recognize and develop multiple aspects for the health components of fitness that will vary depending on one's goals. What was your goal that you wanted to change from Chapter 1? It is important to avoid inactivity and find activities that are enjoyable and likely for you to incorporate into your daily routine and lifestyle. This section will cover two broad areas of physical activity, aerobic or cardiovascular exercise and resistance training exercise to develop muscular strength and muscular endurance.

Cardiovascular Health Guidelines

Aerobic or cardiorespiratory physical activity/exercise is meant for you to elevate your heart rate to a level below its maximum (sub-maximal heart rate) for 30 minutes five times per week for a total of 150 minutes/week at a moderate intensity. Alternatively, smaller 10-minute bouts also show similar improvements in your cardiovascular health if these bouts add up to 30 minutes in one day. In either case, it is important to elevate your heart rate in the range of 40-60% of heart rate reserve (HRR) for moderate intensity (Target Heart Rate Zone). You may also consider vigorous activity (60-85% HRR) for 75 minutes per week. Individuals who find these intensities too challenging may considering beginning at an intensity of 30-40% HRR.

Activity #2: Training Heart Rate Zones Calculation

Calculate your Training Zones using Heart Rate Reserve (HRR).

1) Measure your Resting Heart Rate (RHR) using radial or carotid pulse. Take your pulse with your first two fingers at either radial or carotid arteries.
   - ✓ To find the RADIAL ARTERY, place your fingers (not thumb) on the thumb side of your wrist at the base of your palm. Press gently.
   - ✓ The CAROTID ARTERY is in your neck. Place your first two fingers to the side of your Adam's apple and press gently. Pressing too hard may result in dizziness so just press hard enough to feel the pulse.

   RHR = ________

2) Calculate Maximum Heart Rate (MHR): Select one of the MHR formulas.

   MHR = 220 – Age = ________ OR MHR = 207 – (.7 x Age) = ________

3) Determine moderate intensity (40-60%) Target Heart Rate Zone (THZ)

[(MHR)_____ - _____ (RHR)] x 0.40 + _____ (RHR) = _____ (40% THZ)

[(MHR)_____ - _____ (RHR)] x 0.60 + _____ (RHR) = _____ (60% THZ)

Activity #3: Heart Rate Monitoring

There are two ways to monitor your heart rate (HR):

1) Use your fingers to find your pulse.
2) Wear a heart rate monitor or another wearable that measures HR.

While engaging in physical activity, stop periodically and take either your radial or carotid pulse for 10 seconds. To see if you are in your target heart rate zone (THZ) multiply this number by 6. Or take your range and divide by 6.

Here is an *example*:

- ✓ If your THZ is 140-170 beats per minute, divide 140 and 170 by 6.
- ✓ Your THZ is now 23 - 28 beats in 10 seconds.

Determining if you are in the THZ:

- ✓ If you check your pulse and you count 25 beats during your 10 second count, you are in your zone.
- ✓ If you only count 20 beats, you will want to increase your intensity.
- ✓ If you count 30 beats, you will likely want to decrease your intensity.

Things to Keep in Mind:

- ✓ Some people like to take their pulse for 6 seconds and multiply by 10 as this is easy to do in your head. This works if you are very accurate at taking your pulse. If you are not, and miscount by 1-2 beats, you are multiplying this or by 10.
- ✓ Taking your pulse for more than 10 seconds, results in a less accurate count if you stop moving to take your pulse, as your body will start to recover, and your heart rate will begin to drop after about 15 seconds. Be sure to take your pulse (or check your wearable) periodically during your exercise so that you can adjust your intensity if you are too high or too low.

Activity #4: Heart Rate Monitoring during Activity

Choose one of the following activities: Brisk walking, jogging, dancing or swimming. Complete the activity for a minimum of 10 minutes.

Prior to the start, measure your Heart Rate (HR), then measure your HR again immediately upon stopping the activity.

- ✓ HR before exercise:________
- ✓ HR immediately upon stopping exercise: ________
- ✓ What percentage of your MHR did you reach?
- ✓ Were you in your THZ?

For aerobic activity, the FITT-VP model is helpful in determining and planning your physical activity program. Remember as previously define, the letters stand for: Frequency, Intensity, Time, and Type. Volume and progression have been added to make it FITT-VP. Volume is the product of frequency, intensity, and time. Progression means increasing any one of the FITT components. See below for guidelines for Frequency, Intensity, Time, Type, Volume, and Progression.

Examples of the FITT-VP Model for Aerobic Exercise

FREQUENCY	INTENSITY	TIME	TYPE	VOLUME	PROGRESSION
3-5 days/week	Moderate: 40-60% HRR Vigorous: 60-85% HRR	150 min/wk 75 min/wk	Rhythmic, large muscle groups, running, walking, swimming	Amount FxIxT	Increase by no more than 10%/week, duration before intensity

When performing aerobic exercise, there are three general stages, the warm-up, activity, and cool-down. Prepare your body for the activity by warming up to increase blood flow to your working muscles as well as increase blood flow to your heart. This prepares the body to begin the exercise session and minimizes discomfort. Most warm-ups should generally take 5-15 minutes and be at a slightly lower intensity than the actual exercise session. During the cool-down, the goal is to lower your heart rate to its previous resting level prior to beginning the activity. This prevents blood from pooling in your extremities (which can cause you to feel lightheaded) and allows for a gradual return to rest.

Fitness Walking Technique

It is important to reinforce good mechanics when walking (or running). Poor body posture and leg and arm motions can lead to chronic irritation of the joints and back.

Here are some key tips to think about as you do your brisk walk:

- ✓ Keep your chin level to the ground (many tend to look down).
- ✓ Pull your shoulders down and back but do so in a relaxed vs. stiff manner.
- ✓ Maintain a “proud” chest but don’t overemphasize and arch the back.
- ✓ Lean slightly forward from the hips.
- ✓ Swing your arms in opposition and with the thumbs facing up leading the way.
- ✓ Swing your arms forward and backwards (rather than across the body) allowing the elbows to bend to 90 degrees.
- ✓ Take steps slightly larger than in leisure walking.
- ✓ Place your heel down first and roll through and push off your toes.

Resistance Training Guidelines

While cardiorespiratory exercise improves primarily the cardiovascular system, resistance training primarily improves the muscular system and fitness, which includes muscular strength, muscular endurance, and body composition. The degree to which this is accomplished depends upon the type, intensity, and frequency of resistance training you perform based off your goals (muscular endurance, strength or size).

The American College of Sports Medicine (ACSM) recommends performing resistance training at least twice per week on nonconsecutive days to allow your body to recover. Each session should include 8 to 10 exercises with one set of 8 to 12 repetitions performed for each exercise. The intensity is determined by the percentage of your one-repetition maximum (1-RM). Generally, a beginner should start at approximately 60% of 1-RM which is a weight that you can successfully lift for approximately 15 repetitions to failure (unable to complete another repetition). Generally, weight selection can be based off calculating your 1-RM for an exercise and using the table below (Table 1) as a guideline for the number of repetitions that can be completed at each percentage of 1-RM.

Table 1. Number of Reps Completed to Failure for each %1-RM

% 1-RM	NUMBER OF REPETITIONS COMPLETED TO FAILURE	% 1-RM	NUMBER OF REPETITIONS COMPLETED TO FAILURE
100	1	83	7
95	2	80	8
93	3	77	9
90	4	75	10
87	5	70	12
85	6	65	15

Activity #5: Calculate your 1-RM

Perform an exercise with a weight that is challenging and can be lifted between 5-10 repetitions before reaching failure. Use the following formula to calculate your 1-RM.

1RM = Weight lifted (lbs.) X [1 + (#reps/30)] = ________

*Note #reps are number of repetitions completed to failure (must be ≤ 10)

Source: Epley (1985)

The frequency and intensity (% 1-RM) of resistance training depends on your goals. If your goal is to gain muscle size, also known as hypertrophy, or muscular strength, you would train more often and with greater intensity than if you were training for muscular endurance. Table 2 outlines the guidelines for each goal.

Table 2. Guidelines for Resistance Training Depending on Goal

GOAL	FREQUENCY	INTENSITY	VOLUME
Muscular Endurance	2-3 days/week	≤70% 1-RM	2-4 sets of 10-25 repetitions
Strength (Beginner)	2-3 days/week	60-70% 1-RM	1-3 sets of 8-12 repetitions
Strength (Advanced)	4-5 days/week	≥80%	2-6 sets of 1-8 repetitions
Size (Beginner)	2-3 days/week	60-70% 1-RM	1-3 sets of 8-12 repetitions
Size (Advanced)	4-5 days/week	≥80%	3-6 sets of 6-12 repetitions

Some strategies to use when following guidelines prescribed in Table 2 include performing a set of exercises with a weight that allows you room to complete 1 to 3 more repetitions. This would be the opposite of lifting the weight until failure. This helps prevent overtraining and allows your body to recover for the next workout.

Resistance Training Methods

Resistance training can be carried out in several ways. Often, it's done by performing exercises based on muscle groups, which is one method of training. It can also be accomplished by performing exercises based on movement categories. In this section, you will learn about training using movement pattern categories.

Training using movement patterns is important because it allows optimal balance between each category to minimize risk of injury, especially pushing versus pulling movements. Lower body movement pattern categories include squatting, lunging, hinging, and single-leg exercises; whereas, upper body categories include horizontal pushing and pulling as well as vertical pushing and pulling exercises. Horizontal pushing exercises involve push-ups or bench press variations; whereas, pulling exercises are any type of rowing movement. Vertical pulling exercises include any type of chin-up or pull-up; whereas, pushing exercises involve any type of pressing overhead motion.

Table 3 lists exercises for each category in order of difficulty with the easiest exercises listed first for the movement patterns.

Table 3. Movement Pattern Category Training

UPPER BODY			
HORIZONTAL PULL	**HORIZONTAL PUSH**	**VERTICAL PULL**	**VERTICAL PUSH**
✓ Seated Row ✓ 1-Arm DB Row ✓ Inverted Row	✓ Incline Push-Up ✓ Push-Up ✓ DB Bench Press ✓ BB Bench Press	✓ Lat Pulldown ✓ Chin-Up ✓ Pull-Up	✓ DB Shoulder Press ✓ BB Shoulder Press

LOWER BODY			
SQUAT	LUNGE	HINGE	SINGLE-LEG
✓ BW Squat ✓ Goblet Squat ✓ BB Squat	✓ Split Squat ✓ Reverse Lunge ✓ Forward Lunge	✓ Cable Pull-Through ✓ DB Deadlift ✓ BB Deadlift	✓ Step-Up ✓ SL Romanian DL

BW = bodyweight, **DB** = Dumbbell, **BB** = Barbell, **DL** = Deadlift

Activity #6: Designing a Training Program

It can be overwhelming to design a resistance training program from scratch, and it is generally not recommended. There are three scenarios written below, please choose one option. Once you have chosen an option, you may use the tables on the previous page to help you in selecting exercises; however, it may be useful to explore other resources. If you visit **http://www.exrx.net** you will find a list of exercises based on muscle groups.

- ✓ OPTION A: Choose one exercise from each movement category; perform this routine once per week, 1 set of 8-12 repetitions per exercise.
- ✓ OPTION B**:** Refer to the Two-Day Full Body Routine below (Table 4), select one exercise for each movement category from the previous page; perform this routine twice per week. If you are more advanced, perform 2-3 sets per exercise as opposed to 1 set.
- ✓ OPTION C**:** Write your own 3-day routine. Upon completion, categorize each exercise you have chosen into one of the 8 categories. Are the pushing and pulling movements balanced? Do you include enough variety in the lower body movement categories?

Table 4. Two Day Full Body Movement Pattern Training Routine

DAY OF THE WEEK	
MONDAY	**WEDNESDAY**
Squat	Hip Hinge
Horizontal Push	Horizontal Pull
Lunge	Single-Leg
Vertical Pull	Vertical Push
Core	Core

Flexibility Guidelines

Flexibility training, commonly achieved with stretching exercises, should be completed most days of the week, but at a minimum at least two or three days to see improvements in range of motion. There are several different stretching techniques with static and dynamic stretching being the most commonly used. Dynamic stretches move through a range of motion, while static stretches are held.

Dynamic stretches are usually used to warm up and consist of moving joints through a full range of motion, such as walking lunges and arm circles.

Meanwhile, static stretches are typically performed in the cool down of exercise or physical activity; muscles are warm and thus a greater range of motion can be achieved. Static stretches should be held for a minimum of 10 seconds to allow the muscle to relax and it is preferable to hold the stretch for at least 30 seconds. Stretches should be held to the point of mild discomfort. A good rule of thumb is you should be comfortably uncomfortable and not in pain.

Stability and Functional Movement

Stability is defined as the body's ability to resist a change or disturbance of the body's equilibrium. Being able to stabilize your body is important to both health and sport/recreational activities.

In terms of health, having the musculature to maintain good posture when standing, sitting, and in motion is very important. Stabilization can involve all the muscles in your body, but of importance are the core muscles. These are the muscles between the shoulders and the hips. Weak abdominal and back muscles can lead to low-back pain, and inefficient movement. A strong core allows you to stabilize the trunk, prevent injury, and allow you to produce more efficient arm and leg motions. If you are sitting reading this text, pull in your abs, and pull your shoulders down and back. Feel the difference? A strong core will keep you in this good position.

Activity #7: Core Stability

Stand up and pick up your backpack from the floor with a loose set of abs. Next pull in your abs, stabilize your shoulders, and pick up your backpack.

- ✓ Do you feel a difference?
- ✓ Did you feel stronger the second time?

There are a wide variety of core exercises to choose from and it is good to vary the exercises over time. Here are some suggestions to get started:

- ✓ Plank - knees or toes; hold this position for 10 seconds and gradually work up to 60 seconds. The plank can be performed on the forearms or on the palms with extended arms.
- ✓ Side Plank - knees or toes
- ✓ Bird Dog - one arm or leg at a time, opposing leg and arm same time
- ✓ Dead Dug - one arm or leg at a time, opposing leg and arm same time
- ✓ Medicine Ball Torso Twists standing or in curl-up position

- ✓ Back Extension or Superman Exercise
- ✓ Woodchops (body weight, band, medicine ball)
- ✓ Curl-ups/Crunch - regular, twisting
- ✓ Reverse Crunch

Proper balance between stabilization and mobilization allows for successful bodily movement and plays a part in optimizing success in exercise programs. Muscles can be separated into categories of either stabilizers (ex: rotator cuff) or mobilizers (deltoids). The relationship between stabilizers and mobilizers can either optimize or inhibit activity. Take for example, if your ankle joint is stable, but unable to bend or flex (mobility), it can impose on your natural gait (manner of walking) or ability to squat successfully. If the ankle is unstable and too flexible, injury can occur. Good stability with mobility is what you want. You can achieve this by strengthening stabilizing muscles and stretching properly.

If we are inactive or move with poor technique, our joints lose some of their mobility and stability. Poor posture is a good example of this and becoming more and more prevalent due to constant texting, staring at computer screens, sitting in classes etc. Poor posture puts unnecessary stress on the spine and can lead to back pain. Some signs of poor posture include:

- ✓ Sitting in a slouched position in a chair
- ✓ Leaning far onto a tabletop to gain support while sitting
- ✓ Rounded shoulders
- ✓ Potbelly
- ✓ Back/neck/shoulder pain
- ✓ Head that leans forward or backward

You can counteract poor posture by exercising opposing muscles (your upper back and glutes), strengthening stabilizers, and regularly stretching to ensure joint mobility.

Where and How to Exercise on CCSU's Campus

There are a wide range of opportunities available to you to be more active on campus - both as part of a group or individually.

- ✓ You can join a student club for activities such as Brazilian Jiu-Jitsu, Equestrian Sports, Dance, Fencing, Outdoor Activities, Skiing and much more.

- ✓ The Physical Education & Human Performance Department offers courses in group fitness, yoga and dance including Modern Dance, Ballet, Hip Hop, Afro-Caribbean, and Ballroom Dance. Get fit and get credit at the same time!

- ✓ Visit RECentral (basement level of Kaiser), the recreation department, which staffs the campus fitness facilities, offers group fitness classes, runs intramural sports, and offers fun events designed to bring students together.

Group fitness classes are activities performed with a group of people led by an instructor and accompanied by music. Group fitness classes include Cycling, Zumba®, Cardio, Cardio-kickboxing, HIIT, Water Aerobics, and Yoga. They are fun and motivating and a great way to meet others. All the instructors are used to having beginners join, so if you are a beginner, go a few minutes early and the instructor will help you get started. If you'd rather be playing a sport, round up some friends and sign up for an Intramural Team. The facilities, fitness classes, and other activities are posted on the CCSU RECentral website. Check the schedule and get moving!

Fitness Centers: Where Can I Exercise on Campus?

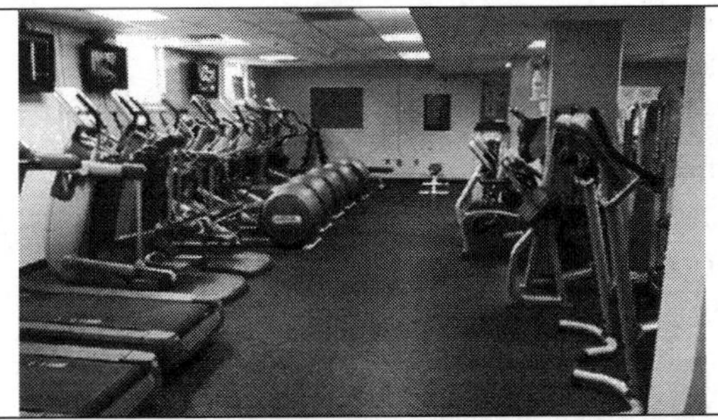

BEECHER FITNESS CENTER

Location: Basement of Beecher Residence Hall
Locker Rooms: Men's and Women's locker rooms are attached to facility

Fitness Equipment: Yoga mats, resistance bands, smart bells, stability balls
Machines: 19 cardio pieces, 6 ellipticals, 2 cross-trainers, 5 treadmills, 3 seated bikes, 3 raised bikes, 18 stack-loaded machines, 8 medicine balls, 2 benches

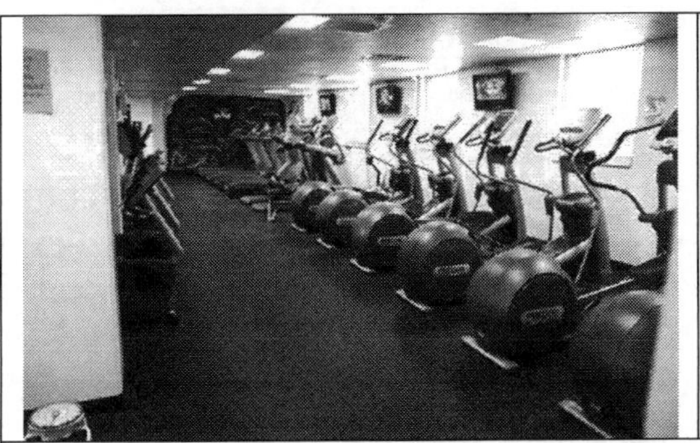

SAM MAY FITNESS CENTER

Location: Basement of Sam May Residence Hall
Locker Rooms: Men's and Women's locker rooms are attached to facility

Fitness Equipment: Yoga mats, resistance bands, smart bells, stability balls
Machines: 19 cardio pieces, 6 ellipticals, 2 cross-trainers, 5 treadmills, 3 seated bikes, 3 raised bikes, 2 benches, 8 medicine balls. 5-75 lb. dumbbells, 18 stack-loaded machines

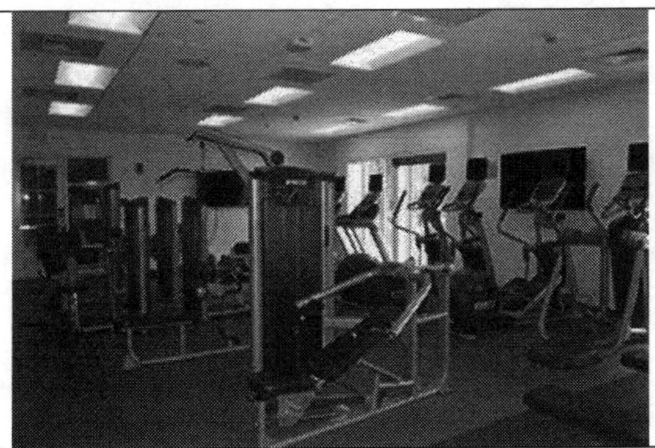

MID CAMPUS FITNESS CENTER

Location: Basement of Mid Campus Residence Hall
Locker Rooms: Men's and Women's locker rooms are attached to facility

Fitness Equipment: Yoga mats, resistance bands
Machines: 9 cardio pieces, 3 ellipticals, 2 cross-trainers, 3 treadmills, 1 seated bike, 1 raised bike, 2 benches

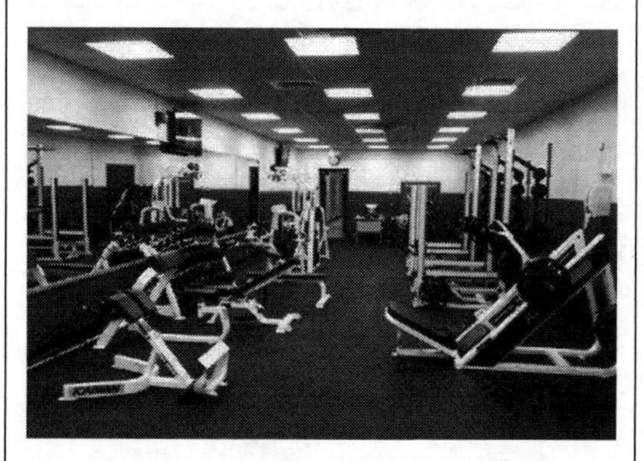

KAISER FITNESS CENTER

Location:
Basement of Kaiser, Room 017
Locker Rooms:
Men's Locker Room is located in Kaiser basement, immediately left of elevator located left of the lobby upon entrance. Women's is located in Kaiser basement, right next to the RECentral Office (044).

Fitness Equipment: Yoga mats, resistance bands, smart bells, stability balls
Machines: 19 cardio pieces, 6 ellipticals, 2 cross-trainers, 5 treadmills, 3 seated bikes, 3 raised bikes, 18 stack-loaded machines, 8 medicine balls, 2 benches

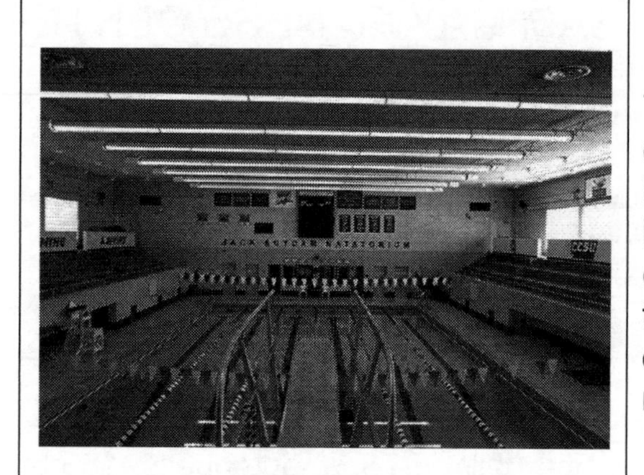

KAISER POOL

To get to the pool in Kaiser Hall you must enter through the Physical Education and Recreation locker rooms located in the basement of Kaiser Hall. There you can change and shower. The entrance is through the showers. All swimmers must enter pool through the associated locker rooms in the basement.

Activity #8: Fitness Center Machine Search!

Visit one of the fitness centers above and use at least 3 pieces of the equipment (cardio machines count). List out the machines you used below.

1)
2)
3)

Activity #9: Attend a Group Fitness Class

Attend one of the group fitness classes provided by RECentral then answer the following questions. For an updated list of classes and times go to the RECentral website: **www.ccsu.edu/recentral/ClassCalendar.html**

1) Which class did you attend and at what time?
2) Did you enjoy the class? Why or why not?
3) Have you ever participated in this type of exercise before?
4) What did you enjoy *most* about this class?
5) What did you enjoy *least* about this class?
6) Do you feel this is something you can incorporate into your weekly schedule? Why or why not?

Chapter Summary

- ✓ Physical wellness and physical activity have many health benefits.
- ✓ Health-related fitness is achieved through developing good levels of cardiorespiratory endurance, muscular strength and endurance, flexibility and body composition.
- ✓ Skill-related fitness enhances performance in sports and recreational activities by achieving agility, balance, coordination, power, reaction time, and speed.
- ✓ Exercise principles and guidelines can help you optimize your fitness goals.
- ✓ Cardiovascular exercise intensity can be monitored using heart rate through taking your pulse or through a heartrate monitor or another wearable.
- ✓ Resistance exercise intensity is measured through percent 1-RM.
- ✓ Core strength and stability helps prevent injury and enhance physical ability.
- ✓ Poor posture can lead to back pain.

Chapter Review Questions

1) Which health-related component of fitness do you feel is the most important?
2) What is the difference between physical activity and exercise?
3) What does a progressive overload look like for aerobic exercise? For muscular strength and/or endurance?
4) Describe the FITT-VP for aerobic exercise.
5) What movement categories should be balanced when designing a resistance training program?
6) How many sets and repetitions should a someone perform if they have never lifted weights before?
7) How long do you hold a static stretch to see benefits?

References

Cooper, K. (1968). A means of assessing maximal oxygen intake correlation between field and treadmill testing. *Journal of the American Medical Association* 203(03), 201-204.

Epley, B. (1985). *Poundage Chart. Boyd Epley Workout.* Lincoln, NE: Body Enterprises.

Exercise Prescription (n.d.). Retrieved from: **http://www.exrx.net**

Centers for Disease Control and Prevention (2009). *Physical Activity.* Retrieved from: **https://www.cdc.gov/healthyplaces/healthtopics/physactivity.htm**

US Department of Health and Human Services (2008). *Physical activity guidelines for Americans, 2008.* **http://www.health.gov/PAGuidelines**.

Chapter 3

Nutritional Wellness

By Cassandra Forsythe York, PhD, RD

Chapter Objectives

After reading this chapter, students should be able to:

- ✓ Understand what nutrition means;
- ✓ Recognize what a healthy diet is made of;
- ✓ Understand components of food and why we eat;
- ✓ Know how to build nutritious meals and snacks;
- ✓ Recognize food for optimal body composition; and
- ✓ Understand what a healthy body is.

What is Good Nutrition?

"Our food should be our medicine, and our medicine should be our food"- Hippocrates

Defining Nutrition

When you read the word 'nutrition', what was the first thing that came to mind? Was it, food? Eating? Diet? Vegetables? Fruit? Health? If it was any of these choices, you would be correct. Nutrition is defined as: *The process of providing or obtaining the food necessary for health and growth.*

It's also simply known as food or nourishment. And, like all things related to our health and bodies, there is "good" nutrition and "bad" nutrition; there's a way of eating and choosing foods that optimizes your health and well-being, while there's another way that diminishes how you feel, and increases your risk of sickness and disease. Most people know what good nutrition is, but many times we have a hard time following a nutritious diet mostly because we don't enjoy nutritious foods, or we don't have access to them (due to lack of resources or finances).

The Truth about Good Nutrition

A comedian once joked that he knew that kale was good for him, but to him, it tasted like what death would taste like if it were a food – of course that got a huge laugh from the audience. He then said that he couldn't give up burgers, fries, and chocolate because they were his favorite foods and he'd rather be unhealthy than eat chicken, kale, and beans. In his mind, and in the minds of most people, good nutrition means eating foods that don't have much flavor and giving up all the comfort foods you love. Even Mark Twain, the famous American author (born 1835, died 1910) wrote,

> *"The only way to keep your health is to eat what you don't want, drink what you don't like, and do what you'd rather not" ~ Mark Twain*

Clearly, choosing good nutrition for good health is something many of us find dissatisfying – and we've felt this way for over a century! However, eating a healthy diet doesn't mean you have to eliminate your favorite foods. Items like French fries and cookies can fit into a healthy eating plan, as long as your diet also includes more traditional healthy foods such as fresh vegetables and fruit, fish and poultry, dairy, and whole grains.

What is a Healthy Diet?

A healthful diet is described as one that is:

- ✓ Adequate
- ✓ Moderate
- ✓ Balanced
- ✓ Nutrient Dense
- ✓ Varied

A diet that is **ADEQUATE** means that it is one that provides enough energy (in the form of calories) and nutrients to support a person's health. However, a diet that is adequate in one area can still be inadequate in another. For example, many people eat more than enough calories, but may not eat enough healthy fat or specific nutrients – this often happens in people who eat a lot of empty calories in the form of junk food without also consuming unprocessed, natural foods.

The amount of any food you eat should be **MODERATE** – not too much and not too little. Ideally you should eat a little bit of everything and not a lot of anything. A healthy diet is one that contains the right amounts of foods for maintaining an ideal weight and optimal health. A moderate diet does include candy and fried foods along with steamed vegetables and lean protein. Having a little bit of everything helps us to find more joy in eating while keeping our health in check.

A **BALANCED** diet is one that contains the right combinations of foods to provide the right proportions of nutrients for your body. Your body needs many types of foods in varying amounts to maintain health, which is why eating a variety of foods from different food groups is ideal.

NUTRIENT-DENSITY means that a food has a high amount of nutrients (vitamins, minerals, phytonutrients), with a low number of calories. Nutrients in foods help us produce energy, fight off diseases, and give us optimal physical and mental health. Examples of nutrient-dense foods include fruits, berries and vegetables, whole grains (oatmeal), and legumes (lentils, soybeans).

Finally, as the famous saying goes, "**VARIETY** is the spice of life" – which is exactly why comfort and junk foods can fit into a healthy diet. Variety refers to eating many different foods from the different food groups on a regular basis. Ideally, we shouldn't eat the same thing every day, although for some people, eating the same things over and over again is easier than cooking many different meals. Not only will this lead to boredom and relapse (falling off the wagon from a healthy diet), your body will miss out on the nutrients found only in specific foods. Since there is not one perfect food, we need a variety of different foods eaten together to supply our bodies with the nutrients we need.

What is an Unhealthy Diet?

An unhealthy diet is any consistent food intake that:

- ✓ promotes unnecessary weight/body fat gain
- ✓ causes gut dysfunction (flatulence, bloating, diarrhea and/or constipation)
- ✓ leads to anxiety or poor sleep
- ✓ initiates allergies, intolerances and/or illnesses
- ✓ makes it hard for you to focus, feel well, and have positive mental clarity

The components of an unhealthy diet are mostly junk foods that are high in sugar, salt and/or fat. They also include sweets, baked goods, fast foods, man-made fats and sugars, sodas and high calorie beverages, and alcoholic drinks.

As you read, these foods can still fit into a healthy diet, but they just can't be everything that you eat. You can't start your day with a fast food breakfast, snack on chocolate bars, soda, and potato chips all day long and still expect to feel good or live healthy.

How to Build a Healthy Diet

Scientists and nutritionists have been studying the effects of food on health for many decades and have come up with Dietary Guidelines for Americans based on this research. Every five years these recommendations are revised by the U.S. government to reflect our current knowledge on nutrition for health. The guidelines are jointly published by the USDA and the Department of Health and Human Service. Key Recommendations of the 2015-2020 Dietary Guidelines are:

- ✓ *A variety of vegetables from all of the subgroups—dark green, red and orange, legumes (beans and peas), and starchy vegetables such as potatoes and turnips*
- ✓ *Fruits, especially whole fruits and berries*
- ✓ *Grains, at least half of which are whole grains (oats, rice, quinoa)*
- ✓ *Fat-free or low-fat dairy, including milk, yogurt, cheese, and/or fortified soy beverages*
- ✓ *A variety of protein foods, including seafood, lean meats and poultry, eggs, legumes (beans and peas), and nuts, seeds, and soy products*
- ✓ *Oils (olive oils, vegetable oils)*

- ✓ *If alcohol is consumed, it should be consumed in moderation—up to one drink per day for women and up to two drinks per day for men—and only by adults of legal drinking age.*
- ✓ ***Consume a healthy eating pattern that accounts for all foods and beverages within an appropriate calorie level for your body.***

In order to you to help you figure out if your daily meals are nutritious and in line with the Dietary Guidelines, use MyPlate – an online tool to help you plan your meals and snacks.

Use MyPlate for Healthy Meals

In 2011, the USDA launched ChooseMyPlate (Figure 1) - a nutritional graphic designed to help Americans easily follow the key recommendations of the current Dietary Guidelines for Americans. It replaces the former Food Pyramid previously used to help people follow a better diet.

This graphic, shown below, consists of a place setting with a plate and glass divided into the five major food groups: vegetables, fruits, grains, dairy and protein. It's supplemented with additional recommendations, such as "Make half your plate fruits and vegetables", "Switch to 1% or skim milk", "Make at least half your grains whole", and "Vary your protein food choices". The guidelines also recommend portion control while still enjoying food, as well as reductions in sodium and sugar intakes.

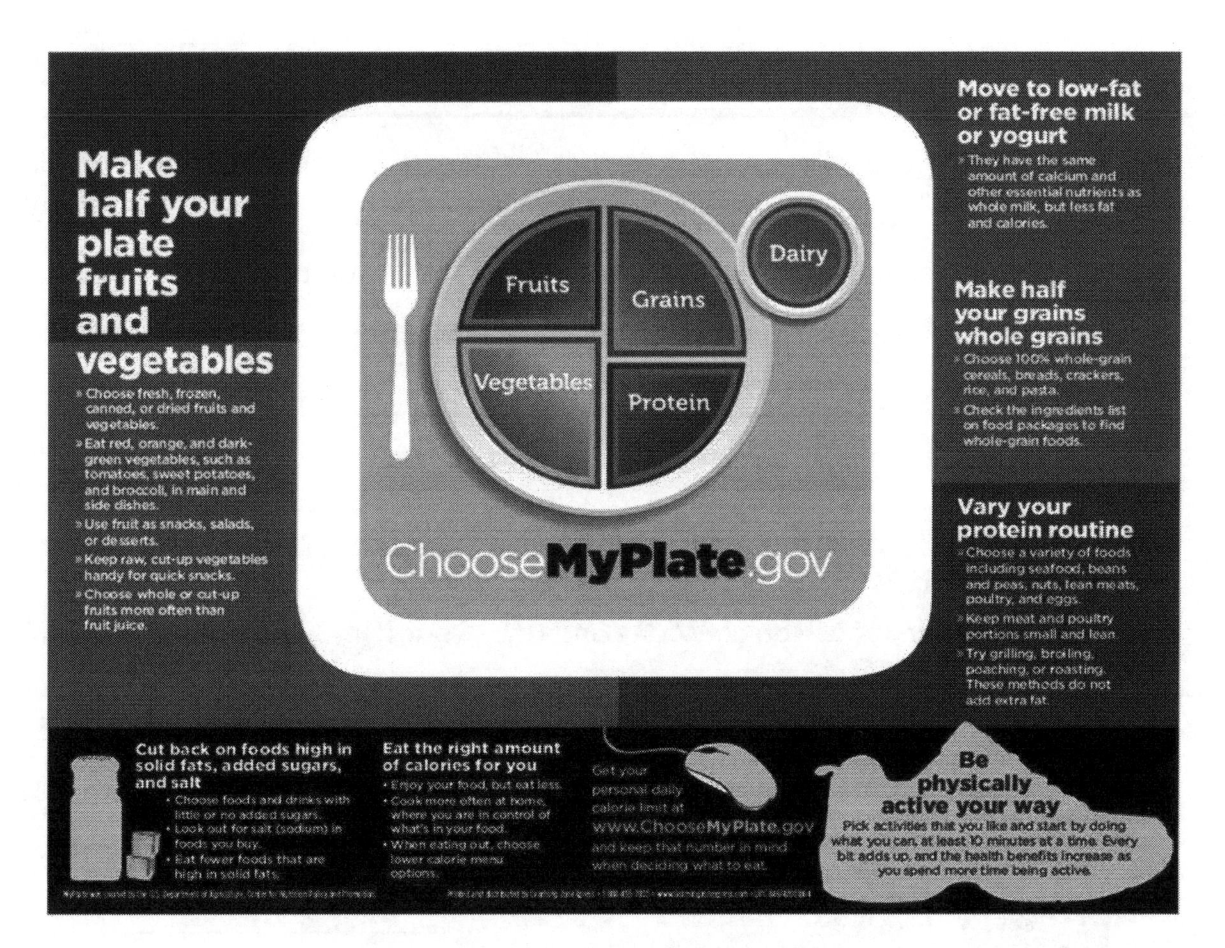

Figure 1. MyPlate Recommendations

After looking at this plate, as yourself the following questions?

- ✓ Do all your meals and snacks contain a fruit or a vegetable?
- ✓ Do they contain whole grains and protein?
- ✓ Do you consume any dairy?

Thankfully, not all your meals have to contain each of these, but your day should have the recommended amounts of each of the five major food groups.

Activity #1: MyPlate Assessment

To see if your overall daily diet meets the recommendations, fill out the MyPlate Daily Checklist worksheet below (Figure 2). This worksheet is based on an intake of 2000 calories per day; your exact needs may be higher or lower. For your own worksheet that matches your caloric needs, please visit:

www.choosemyplate.gov/MyPlate-Daily-Checklist

MyPlate Daily Checklist

Write down the foods you ate today and track your daily MyPlate, MyWins!

Food group targets for a 2,000 calorie* pattern are:		Write your food choices for each food group	Did you reach your target?
Fruits	**2 cups** 1 cup of fruits counts as • 1 cup raw or cooked fruit; or • 1/2 cup dried fruit; or • 1 cup 100% fruit juice.		Y N
Vegetables	**2 1/2 cups** 1 cup vegetables counts as • 1 cup raw or cooked vegetables; or • 2 cups leafy salad greens; or • 1 cup 100% vegetable juice.		Y N
Grains	**6 ounce equivalents** 1 ounce of grains counts as • 1 slice bread; or • 1 ounce ready-to-eat cereal; or • 1/2 cup cooked rice, pasta, or cereal.		Y N
Protein	**5 1/2 ounce equivalents** 1 ounce of protein counts as • 1 ounce lean meat, poultry, or seafood; or • 1 egg; or • 1 Tbsp peanut butter; or • 1/4 cup cooked beans or peas; or • 1/2 ounce nuts or seeds.		Y N
Dairy	**3 cups** 1 cup of dairy counts as • 1 cup milk; or • 1 cup yogurt; or • 1 cup fortified soy beverage; or • 1 1/2 ounces natural cheese or 2 ounces processed cheese.		Y N

Figure 2. MyPlate Daily Checklist

There are other versions of MyPlate to help guide people with different dietary choices. For example, there is the MyPlate for Vegetarians (Figure 3).

COOPERATIVE EXTENSION SERVICE
UNIVERSITY OF KENTUCKY COLLEGE OF AGRICULTURE, FOOD AND ENVIRONMENT, LEXINGTON, KY 40546

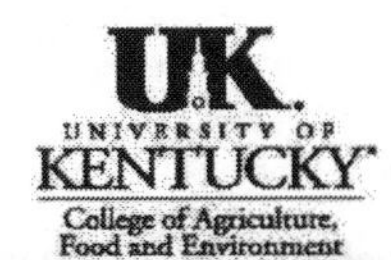

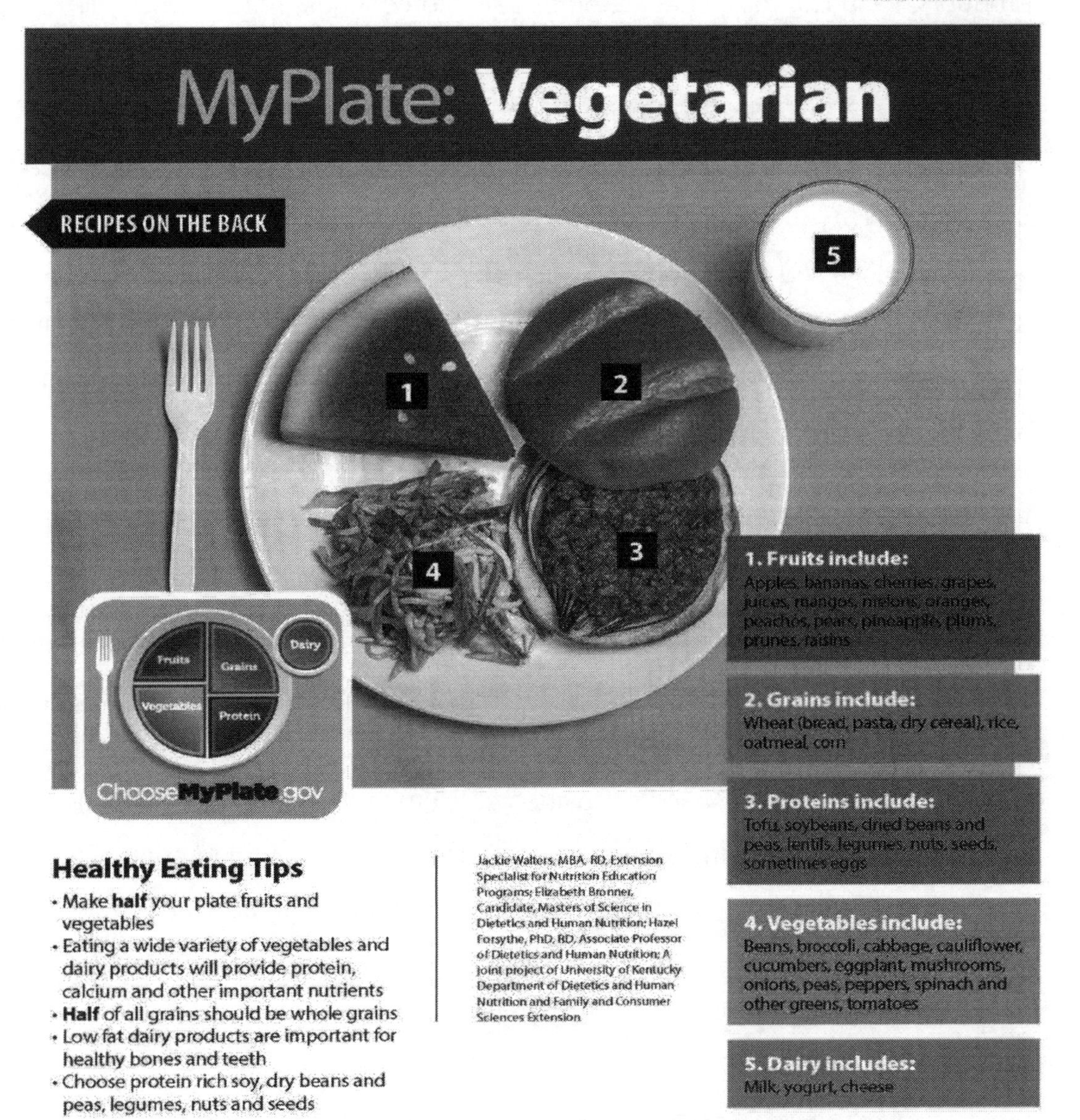

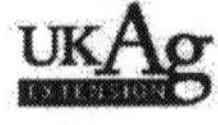

Agriculture and Natural Resources • Family and Consumer Sciences • 4-H Youth Development • Community and Economic Development

Figure 3. MyPlate for Vegetarians

Vegetarianism in a Nutshell

The basics: Vegetarians do not eat meat, fish, and poultry. Some vegetarians eat eggs and/or dairy. Vegans are vegetarians who abstain from eating or using all animal products, including milk, cheese, other dairy items, eggs, honey, wool, silk, or leather.

Among the many reasons for being a vegetarian are health, environmental, and ethical concerns; dislike of meat; non-violent beliefs; compassion for animals; and economics. The Academy of Nutrition and Dietetics has affirmed that a vegetarian diet can meet all known nutrient needs. The key to a healthy vegetarian diet, as with any other diet, is to eat a wide variety of foods, including fruits, vegetables, plenty of leafy greens, whole grain products, nuts, seeds, and legumes, and the right amount of foods to meet your calorie needs. Limit your intake of sweets and fatty foods.

Here are tips to help you make good vegetarian-based food choices:

- ✓ Build meals around protein sources that are naturally low in fat, such as beans, lentils, and rice. Don't overload meals with high-fat cheeses to replace the meat.
- ✓ Calcium-fortified soymilk provides calcium in amounts similar to milk.
- ✓ Many Asian and Indian restaurants offer a variety of vegetarian dishes.
- ✓ Many foods that typically contain meat or poultry can be made vegetarian. This can increase vegetable intake and cut unhealthy fat intake. Consider:
  - pasta primavera or pasta with marinara or pesto sauce
  - veggie pizza
  - vegetable lasagna
  - tofu-vegetable stir fry
  - bean burritos or tacos
- ✓ Add vegetarian meat substitutes to soups and stews to boost protein without adding saturated fat or cholesterol. These include tempeh (cultured soybeans with a chewy texture), tofu, or wheat gluten (seitan).

- ✓ For barbecues, try veggie burgers, soy hot dogs, marinated tofu or tempeh, and veggie kabobs.
- ✓ Make bean burgers, lentil burgers, or pita halves with falafel (spicy ground chickpea patties).
- ✓ Most restaurants can accommodate vegetarian modifications to menu items by substituting meatless sauces, omitting meat from stir-fries, and adding vegetables or pasta in place of meat. These substitutions are more likely to be available at restaurants that make food to order.

The Harvard Healthy Eating Plate

Another infographic tool to help you eat better is the Harvard Healthy Eating Plate (Figure 4). This tool was created by nutrition experts at Harvard School of Public Health and editors at Harvard Health Publications, to address deficiencies in the USDA's MyPlate. The Healthy Eating Plate provides detailed guidance, in a simple format, to help people make the best eating choices.

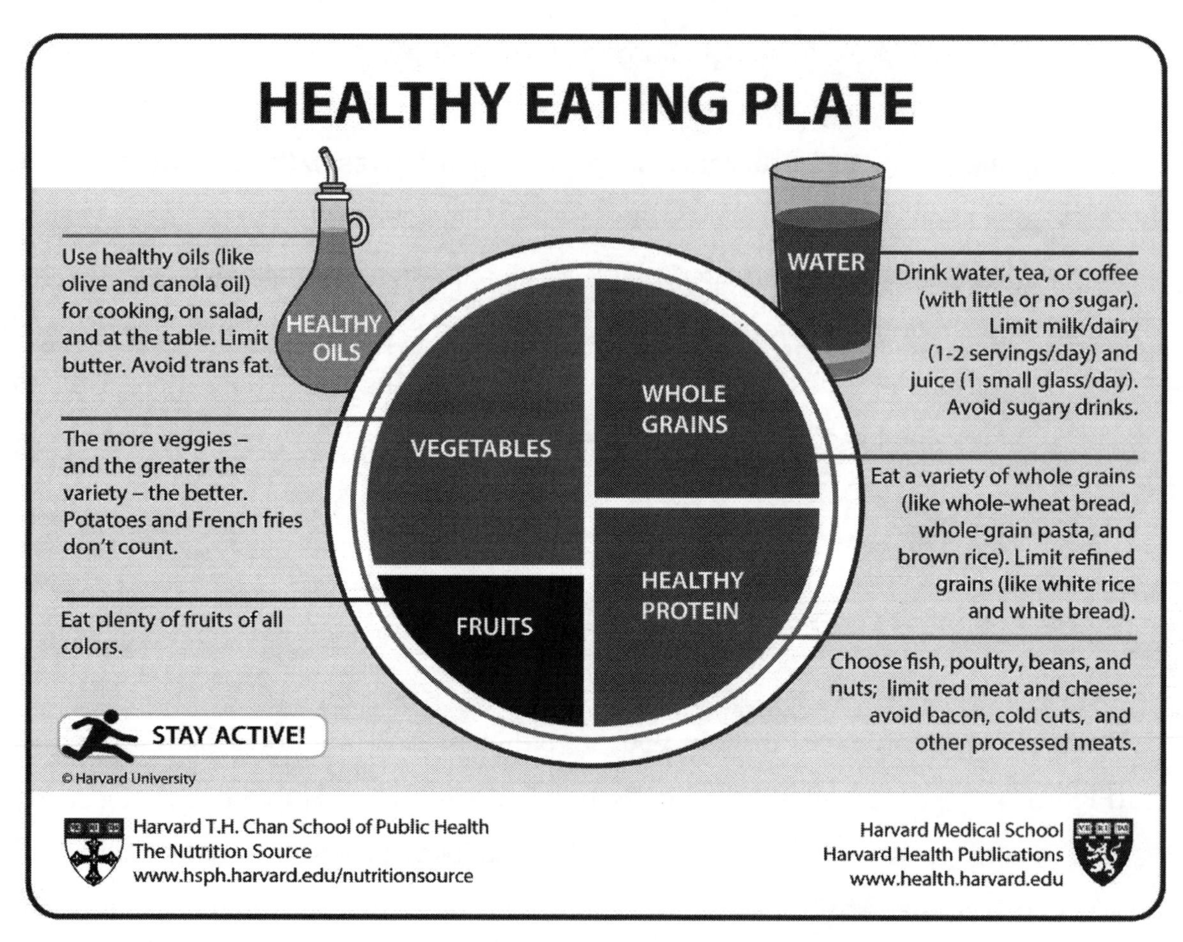

Figure 4. The Harvard Healthy Eating Plate

No matter which tool you choose to follow, choose the one that helps you select good nutrition choices each day. If you need extra help with meal planning or dietary choices, reach out to a Registered Dietitian (RD), who is an expert trained to help you with all your nutrition needs.

Examples of Quick and Healthy Meals and Snacks

Use the images in the picture below to help you plan your next meal or snack. Each contains a fruit or vegetable, a source of protein, and natural sources of healthy fats.

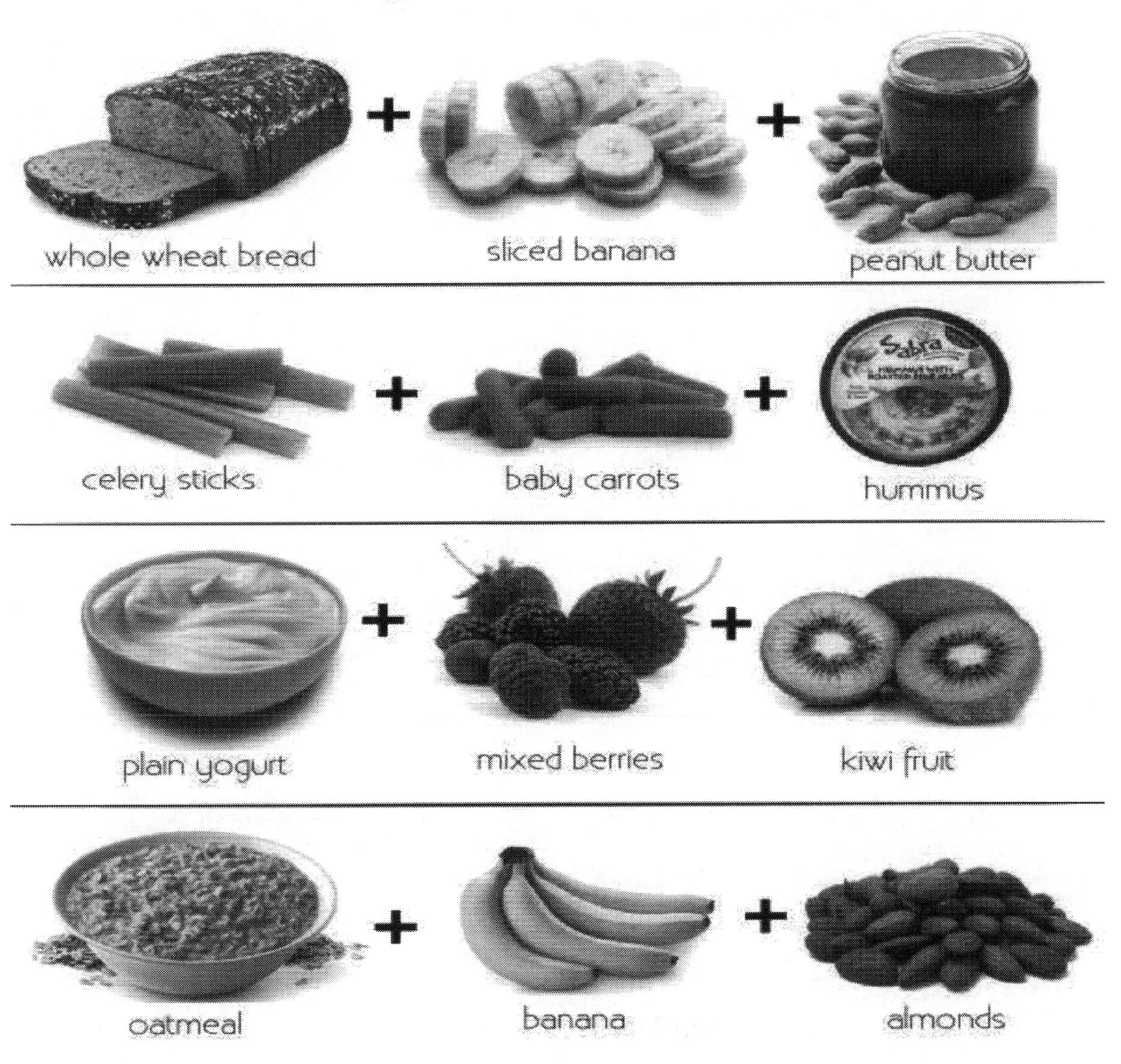

Why Do We Eat?

People eat for a number of reasons. Some eat because they are hungry, some have an emotional attachment to eating, and other people just can't restrain themselves when they see a certain food. The list of motives behind why people actually eat can go on and on. However, all these reasons usually will fall into two main categories; eating for enjoyment and eating for nourishment.

When we eat for enjoyment, we aren't filling any biological need, other than satisfying desire. Eating for nourishment, on the other hand, is the body's way of providing itself with the essential nutrients and energy it needs for growth and survival. Of the nutrients you need, there are *major* nutrients and *minor* nutrients.

What Is Food Made Of?

The major essential nutrients you need every day include carbohydrates, proteins, fats, and water, which are required in large amounts, and, other than water, provide our body with energy (in the form of calories).

The minor nutrients are required in lesser amounts and include vitamins and minerals and other nutrients that help our body make energy (they don't provide any energy though) and prevent diseases.

We also choose foods based on economic and environmental influences: what foods we can afford, what we have available to us in stores and dining halls, and what we feel comfortable with based on our experiences growing up and the influences of our parents. Regardless of the influences that external factors have on our food choices, we eat to give our body the fuel it needs to function normally.

The following describes what food is made of and what benefit it has on our body.

Carbohydrates for Energy and Fiber

Carbohydrates, which include fiber, starch, and sugars are found in many of the foods we eat, primarily fruits, vegetables, and grains (pasta, breads, whole grains). Dairy, legumes, nuts, and seeds contain carbohydrates too, but they also contain protein and fats. These carbohydrates are high quality and should be eaten often. Low quality carbohydrate foods include sodas, sweets, sugary cereals, sports drinks and most junk food – choose these least often (Figure 5).

High Quality Carbohydrate Foods – Eat Most Often

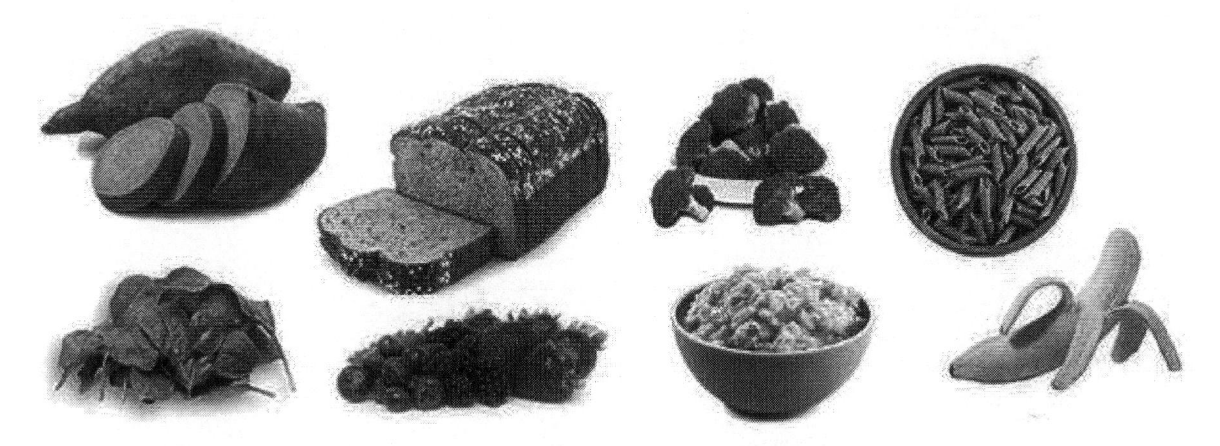

Low Quality Carbohydrate Foods – Eat Least Often

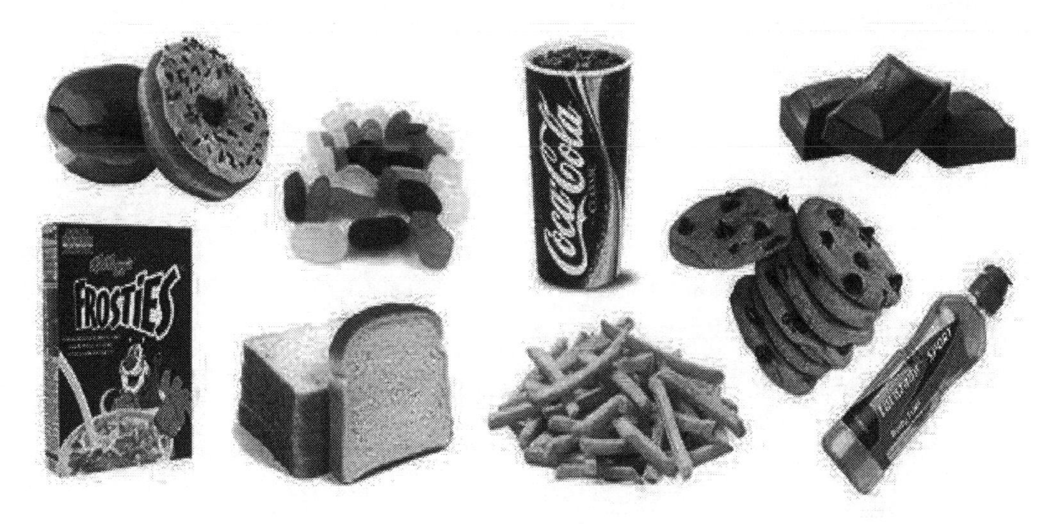

Figure 5. High- and Low-Quality Carbohydrate Foods

We eat foods rich in carbohydrates because they are one of our body's main food sources of energy. The digestive system breaks down most carbohydrates (other than fiber) into a simple sugar called glucose. Glucose is the most important source of energy for your body. It's stored in the liver and muscle as glycogen and floats around in your body as blood glucose (or blood sugar). Fiber can't be broken down by the digestive system but is important because it helps move waste through the intestinal tract, lowers cholesterol levels in the blood (by binding to fat in the intestine), and provides energy for the good bacteria living in your colon. Beans are a great source of fiber, with the average cup of beans providing 14 grams of fiber. Dry roasted soybeans provide the most fiber with 30 grams per cup, and Navy beans have 19 grams in a single cup cooked. You can get more fiber in your diet by adding beans to your meals (sprinkled on salads or eaten as a side dish) or by choosing whole grains like oatmeal for breakfast which has about 4 grams of fiber per serving (half Cup cooked).

Protein Power

Proteins are primarily found in meats, fish, poultry, and dairy, but are also found in non-animal sources such as beans/legumes (soybeans), grains (quinoa), nuts (peanut butter), and seeds (Figure 6).

We eat protein because it provides building blocks for the variety of different proteins in our bodies including our muscle, enzymes, blood proteins (i.e., hemoglobin) and hormones. Protein alone doesn't provide our body with much usable energy –we prefer to use protein-rich foods to build protein in our body. However, many protein foods are also a source of healthy dietary fats and carbohydrates. Try to avoid protein foods that are deep fried (fish sticks or chicken fingers) or preserved with sodium nitrite (deli meats and sausages) and instead choose proteins from the sources pictured below.

High Quality Protein Foods

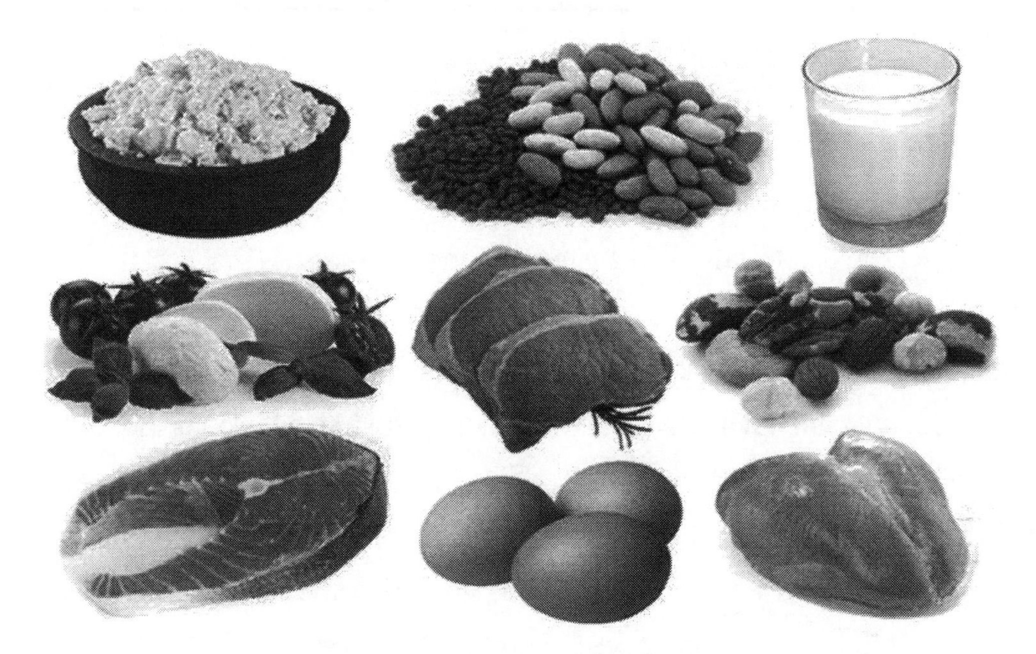

Figure 6. Protein Foods

The building blocks of proteins are known as amino acids; there are 20 amino acids that provide the raw material for all proteins. Nine are essential, meaning our body cannot make them, we must get them from food. This is why you must eat foods rich in protein—to take in all the essential amino acids. Because the body does not store amino acids like it does carbohydrates and fats, you need to eat protein every day. Essential amino acids are only found in animal products – these protein sources are called Complete Proteins. Grains, beans, and nuts are lacking in one of more of the essential amino acids and are therefore called Incomplete Proteins.

Vegetarian Proteins

If you choose to not eat animal products (because you are following a vegetarian or vegan diet) make sure you are consuming a variety of vegetable (incomplete) protein sources to get all the essential amino acids. Vegetable sources of protein such as beans and whole grains are good choices, and they offer fiber, vitamins, and minerals. See the MyPlate for Vegetarians Guidelines earlier in this chapter for more information.

Facts about Fats

Fats are often feared because many people equate dietary fat to body fat, or to heart disease. However, not all fats are bad. In fact, many fats from whole food sources provide your body with essential fats (ones your body cannot make, but needs for health), in addition to fat-soluble vitamins and minerals.

Nutritious sources of fat include nuts, seeds, oils, eggs, fish, and meat. Eggs are vilified because the fat in the yolks (specifically the cholesterol) is thought to contribute to high blood cholesterol levels, which may lead to heart disease. However, egg yolks in moderation are actually beneficial to heart health and provide important nutrients for eye and brain health. Saturated fat, found in meats and dairy, is also not as detrimental to health as was once thought.

The most evil fats are the *trans* fatty acids. These fats are made by humans through a process known as hydrogenation. To avoid these fats, read ingredient labels on foods and watch out for the words “hydrogenated” or “partially-hydrogenated”. See the following infographic for more information (Figure 7).

Trans Fat

Nutrition Facts

Serving Size 1 package (272g)
Servings Per Container 1

Amount Per Serving	
Calories 300	Calories from Fat 45
	% Daily Value*
Total Fat 5g	**8%**
Saturated Fat 1.5g	**8%**
Trans Fat 0g	
Cholesterol 30mg	**10%**
Sodium 430mg	**18%**
Total Carbohydrate 55g	**18%**
Dietary Fiber 6g	**24%**
Sugars 23g	
Protein 14g	
Vitamin A	80%
Vitamin C	35%
Calcium	6%
Iron	15%

*Percent Daily Values are based on a 2,000 calorie diet. Your Daily Values may be higher or lower depending on your calorie needs:

	Calories:	2,000	2,500
Total Fat	Less than	65g	80g
Saturated Fat	Less than	20g	25g
Cholesterol	Less than	300mg	300mg
Sodium	Less than	2,400mg	2,400mg
Total Carbohydrate		300g	375g
Dietary Fiber		25g	30g

Trans fat can increase the risk of developing cardiovascular disease.

***Trans* fat is a nutrient to get less of.**

Update on *Trans* Fat

On June 16, 2015, the U.S. Food and Drug Administration (FDA) took action that will significantly reduce the use of partially hydrogenated oils, the major source of artificial *trans* fats in the food supply. This action is expected to reduce cardiovascular disease and prevent thousands of fatal heart attacks each year in the U.S.

FDA is providing companies three years to either reformulate products without partially hydrogenated oils and/or petition FDA to permit specific uses. Food companies have already been working to remove partially hydrogenated oils from processed foods and FDA anticipates that many may eliminate them ahead of the three-year compliance date.

It's important to note that *trans* fat will not be completely gone from foods because it occurs *naturally* in small amounts in meat and dairy products, and is present at very low levels in other edible oils.

http://www.fda.gov/nutritioneducation

What It Is

Trans fat is an unsaturated fat, but it is structurally different than unsaturated fat that occurs naturally in plant foods. *Trans* fat has **detrimental health effects** and is not essential in the diet.

There are **two sources** of *trans* fat:

- ***Trans* fat formed naturally** – this type of *trans* fat is produced in the gut of some grazing animals (such as cattle and sheep).
- ***Trans* fat formed artificially during food processing** – this type of *trans* fat is created during a process called "partial hydrogenation" in which hydrogen is added to liquid vegetable oil to make it more solid, and therefore more resistant to becoming spoiled or rancid. The process generally does not make the oil completely solid, resulting in "partially" hydrogenated oils.

Where It Is Found

***Trans* fat formed naturally** is found in small amounts in some animal products, such as meats and dairy products.

***Trans* fat formed artificially during food processing** is found in partially hydrogenated oils used in a variety of foods, including:

- Coffee creamer
- Fast food
- Frozen pizza
- Grain-based desserts (such as cakes, cookies, and frozen pies)
- Ready-to-use frostings
- Refrigerated dough products (such as biscuits and cinnamon rolls)
- Savory snacks (such as crackers and microwave popcorn)
- Vegetable shortening and stick margarine

What It Does

Partially hydrogenated oils are used by food manufacturers to improve the texture, shelf life, and flavor stability of foods. Partially hydrogenated oils should not be confused with "fully hydrogenated oils," which are solid fats that contain very low levels of *trans* fat.

Trans Fat 1

Figure 7. All about Trans Fats

The role of dietary fats in the body are to:

- ✓ balance good and bad cholesterol levels,
- ✓ serve a structural role in making and repairing cells
- ✓ help carry other nutrients throughout the bloodstream

Fats also provide taste and mouth feel (the food is enjoyable in your mouth) to foods, which makes them more satiating - and can help you eat less! Just like carbohydrates, there are high quality fats and low-quality fats. We want to emphasize high quality fats in our meals and minimize the low-quality choices (Figure 8).

High-Quality Fat Foods vs Low-Quality Fat Foods

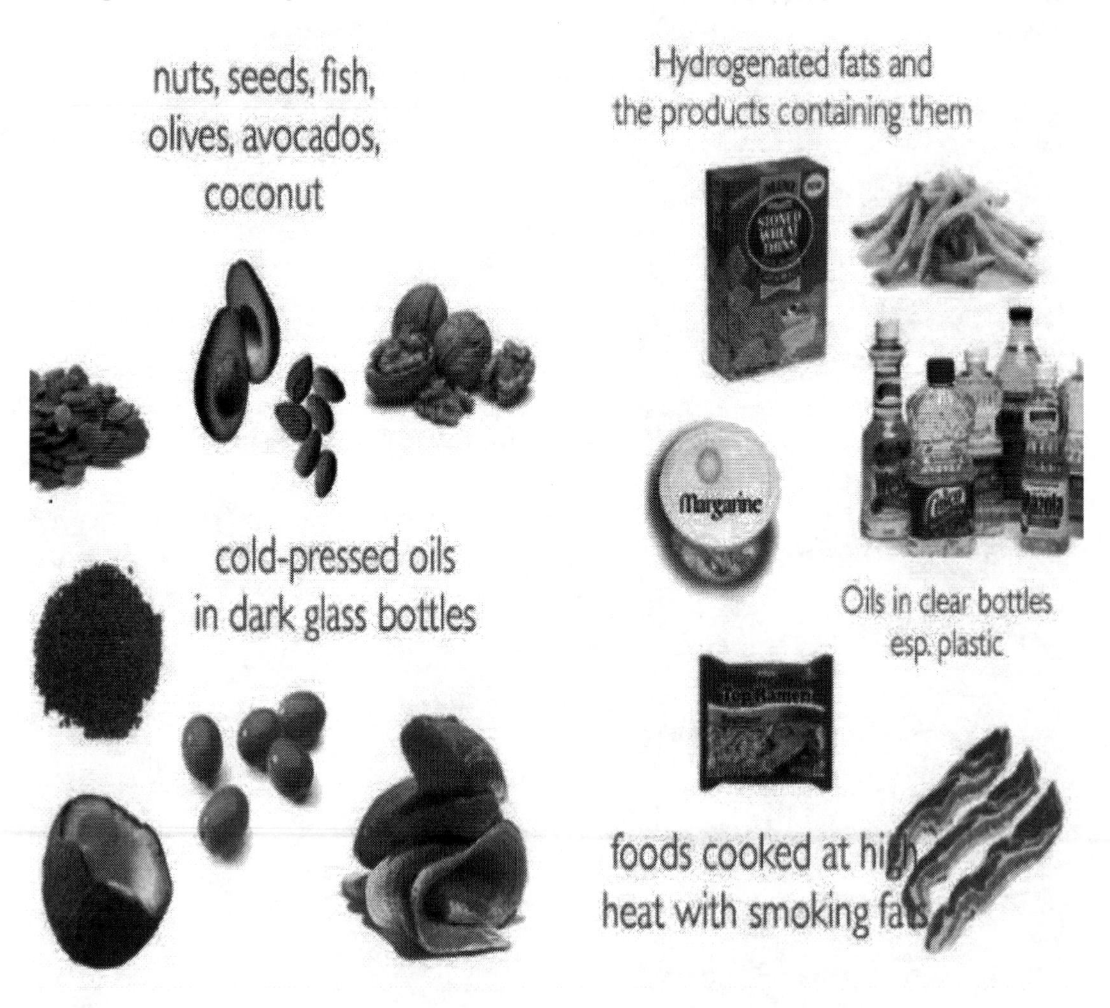

Figure 8. High- and Low-Quality Fat Foods

Fats are made up of fatty acids, which include saturated, monounsaturated and polyunsaturated fatty acids. The essential fats from foods include the omega-3 and omega-6 polyunsaturated fatty acids and are found in fish such as salmon and trout; nuts, such as walnuts and pumpkin seeds; and oils, such as flaxseed oil. We need these fats to help our bodies grow and repair themselves properly; they are also needed to lower our chances of developing heart disease, reduce our risk of inflammatory disorders like arthritis, and prevent a decline in cognitive function and mental health. The omega-3 fats from fish are so important that the American Heart Association recommends eating fish (particularly fatty fish) at least two times (two servings) a week. Each serving is 3.5 ounce cooked, or about ¾ cup of flaked fish. Fatty fish like salmon, mackerel, herring, lake trout, sardines, and albacore tuna are high in omega-3 fatty acids.

How much Protein, Carbohydrates, and Fat Should You Eat Each Day?

Your requirements for these major nutrients depend on your total calorie intake – which is the amount of energy you need each day to maintain your activity levels while preventing unnecessary fat gain (from excessive food intake), or muscle loss (from undereating). Since your calorie requirements may change from day-to-day depending on what you do for exercise, and sometimes hormonal swings, aim for a percentage range of protein, carbohydrates, and fat instead of counting grams of these macronutrients. For good health, these are the ideal recommendations:

- ✓ **PROTEIN** 20-35% of total caloric intake from animal and vegetable sources.
- ✓ **CARBOHYDRATES** 40-50% of total caloric intake primarily from vegetables, legumes, whole grains, and fruits (in order of amounts eaten)
- ✓ **FAT** 20-30% of total caloric intake from unprocessed, natural sources (egg yolks, salmon, nuts, avocado, cheese, hummus), and oils (olive oil, coconut oil, butter, fish oil, flax oil).

How Many Calories Should You Eat?

Calories have (jokingly) been defined as:

<u>CALORIES</u> /ˈkal(ə)rē/ (noun) – *Tiny creatures that live in your closet and sew your clothes a little bit tighter every night*

Calories are, in fact, units of energy found in food; they are the reasons why we eat – to obtain the fuel needed for our bodies to grow, repair and reproduce. Every person has an ideal number of calories (energy) they should eat each day to maintain a healthy body and support activity levels. When we eat too many calories, we gain weight and may increase our risk of diseases. When we eat too few calories, we will lose weight, and may also increase our risk of diseases. The goal to to find caloric balance for your needs, and it changes depending on several factors including:

- ✓ Activity level
- ✓ Illness or disease
- ✓ Hormone fluctuations
- ✓ Level of muscle in your body

Scientists have explored the determination of calorie needs in humans for centuries and have come up with several different ways for us to figure out what we need. The most common metabolic equation to determine the level of calories you should eat each day is the Harris-Benedict equation. You can find many websites online that have a Harris-Benedict calculator available, that allows you to input your current height, weight and activity level to figure out your daily caloric needs.

However, even with a calorie goal in mind, counting calories is not an accurate science. There are many reasons why you may over-estimate or under-estimate your caloric intake, which is why counting calories can only be considered an estimation – not an exact method. Also, counting daily calories may lead to eating disorders and obsessions with food (or the lack of it). As such, it's ideal to build your daily intake off a healthy plate, as described earlier in this chapter, by incorporating all the five major food groups, paired with an adequate intake of water and fluids.

Wonderful Water

Water is so important that within just three days without it or any other fluids, you would perish. You can live up to 3 weeks without any food (as long as you had water), but it wouldn't be very enjoyable. More than half of your body weight is from water. This water is needed for you to maintain your body temperature, support blood circulation, excrete waste, and help you digest and absorb nutrients.

Your body loses water throughout the day in urine, sweat, respiration, and other metabolic processes. If you don't consume enough you can become dehydrated, causing symptoms such as headaches, tiredness and loss of concentration. Chronic dehydration can also contribute to a number of health problems, such as constipation and kidney stones.

How Much Water Do You Need?

You may have heard that you should drink eight, 8 oz. glasses of water each day to maintain proper fluid balance. If a person did this, they would take in 64 oz. of water in one day, or about 2 liters. New recommendations from the Institute of Medicine (IOM), recommend that healthy adults, aged 31 to 70 years of age, living in temperate climates consume the following amounts each day:

- **MEN:** 125 oz. (3.7 liters) water per day from all dietary sources
- **WOMEN:** 91 oz. (2.7 liters) water per day from all dietary sources

When the temperature soars, or if you sweat a lot when you exercise, you will need more water each day than this. Aim for an extra 8 oz. (250 ml) at least.

Activity #2: Monitor Your Water Intake

Monitor how much water you drink in one day. For every 8oz of water you consume check off one glass, then answer the questions below.

1. How many total cups (8 oz) of water did you drink? ___________
2. Did you meet your water intake recommendations for today? _________
3. If not, how many ounces were you short? ___________
4. Did you drink water in the morning? ___________
5. Did you drink water before each meal? ___________
6. If you ate a snack did you drink water with that snack? ___________
7. If you exercised, did you drink water before/after your workout? _________

What If You Don't Like Drinking Water?

The recommendations given by the IOM are much more than the former 64 oz. you may have heard about. The thought of drinking this much water might make you feel sick to your stomach, but remember that your total water intake comes from all of the following sources:

- ✓ Drinks, either plain water or as part of other beverages or fluids including tea, coffee, juice, and soups
- ✓ Solid foods, especially fruit (watermelon) and vegetables—even foods such as bread and cheese provide small amounts of fluid

So, if you don't like drinking water, you can still meet some of your water needs through other beverages (like coffee), and high water-containing foods (like fruits and vegetables). Food provides about 20% of your total water needs each day. That means that you'll need to drink at least 2 to 3 liters (~64 oz.) each day of some type of water-containing beverage. Thus, the general recommendation of eight, 8 oz. glasses of fluid is pretty close to being correct.

Vitamins and Minerals

We don't eat vitamins and minerals directly – they are found naturally in the foods we eat in combination with the macronutrients and other micronutrients. For example, dairy is a good source of the mineral calcium, but it's also where we get protein, carbohydrates, and some fat. A healthy balanced diet provides most of the vitamins your body needs. Taking large doses of vitamin supplements can harm your body (although consuming excess vitamins or minerals from foods will not cause harm). Conversely, not getting enough of the right kinds of vitamins or minerals in your diet can lead to health problems.

Vitamins are organic substances made by plants and animals, which are then eaten by humans. There are 13 vitamins: vitamins A, C, D, E, K, and the B vitamins (thiamin, riboflavin, niacin, pantothenic acid, biotin, vitamin B6, vitamin B12, and folate). You can get all your vitamins from the foods you eat, but your body also makes vitamins D and K (it makes vitamin D in the skin and vitamin K in the gut; your body cannot make any of the other vitamins).

Minerals are inorganic substances that are not made by living things. Instead, they are found naturally in soil and water and are absorbed by plants, which are then eaten by people and other animals. Examples of minerals are iron, calcium, and potassium.

Most Americans get the recommended amounts of most vitamins and minerals to meet their needs. However, many people do not get the recommended levels of some important micronutrients. These nutrients are considered to be "nutrients of public health concern" because low intakes are associated with potential health risks and include:

- ✓ Calcium
- ✓ Iron (of concern for young children, pregnant women, and women capable of becoming pregnant who are premenopausal)
- ✓ Potassium
- ✓ Vitamin D

CALCIUM is important for blood clotting, bone and teeth formation, muscle contraction and nervous system function, among other things. Good food sources of calcium include dairy products, fortified cereals and juices, fortified soy milk, green vegetables (spinach, kale and broccoli), and canned seafood with bones. The recommended intake for calcium is 1000 mg per day. You can use food labels to help you choose high calcium foods.

IRON is necessary for growth and development, immune function, red blood cell formation, and wound healing. People who are low in iron feel tired and lethargic. Those most at risk for low iron are athletes and menstruating women. Animal foods (meats, poultry, and seafood) are the best sources of iron. If you avoid animal foods, you can also find iron in beans and peas, dark green vegetables, prunes and prune juice, and fortified foods. Vegetarian sources of iron are best absorbed with a food source of vitamin C, such as red bell peppers, tomatoes, strawberries, or oranges.

POTASSIUM is needed to help regulate blood pressure, maintain proper fluid balance in the body, assist in muscle contraction and nervous system function, and growth and development. Foods rich in potassium include bananas, milk, oranges and orange juice, potatoes and sweet potatoes, spinach, tomatoes, white beans and yogurt.

VITAMIN D, also known as the sunshine vitamin, is made in our skin when we are exposed to the sun. It is necessary for bone growth, calcium balance, hormone production, immune function and blood pressure regulation. Mental health (depression and anxiety) as well as athletic performance is also related to vitamin D levels in the body. The reason why many Americans fall short of vitamin D intake is because few foods are naturally high in Vitamin D – eggs and fish are two of the only sources. As such, many foods are fortified with Vitamin D, and you should seek these out. Otherwise, supplementation may be necessary.

To Supplement or Not?

Dietary supplements are any non-food product that contains a "dietary ingredient" intended to add further nutritional value to (supplement) the diet. A "dietary ingredient" may be one, or any combination, of the following substances:

- ✓ a vitamin
- ✓ a mineral
- ✓ an herb or other botanical
- ✓ an amino acid
- ✓ a dietary substance for use by people to supplement the diet by increasing the total dietary intake
- ✓ a concentrate, metabolite, constituent, or extract

You would only need to add dietary supplements to your daily routine if you specifically knew you were lacking in one nutrient or another. To truly know if you are lacking in a nutrient, a blood test can be taken and reviewed by your physician. Calcium may be low in your diet if you avoid dairy products. Or, if you follow a vegetarian lifestyle, you may lack vitamin B12. Only add supplements to your diet if you really need them and if they were recommended by your physician or RD. Otherwise, they are a waste of money, and they will never compensate for an unhealthy, unbalanced, diet.

Another concern regarding dietary supplements is safety (Figure 9). The laws in the United States regarding dietary supplements are found in the Dietary Supplement Health Education Act of 1994 (DSHEA). This law made it so supplement companies do not have to provide any evidence that their products are safe or effective before they are sold. There is no pre-sale approval process for dietary supplements as there are with pharmaceuticals. Any claims made by a supplement company do not have to be supported by any evidence. The exception to this is if a company sells a "new dietary ingredient" – one that was not sold in the U.S. before 1994. In this case, a supplement company does have to provide some form of evidence that the ingredient is safe for human consumption, however they still do not have to provide evidence that the product works. Most dietary supplements are safe when used as directed, but some can cause adverse reactions ranging from rashes, to gastro-intestinal problems to death. Check with your healthcare provider before taking any dietary supplement and disclose any supplement use when seeking medical treatment.

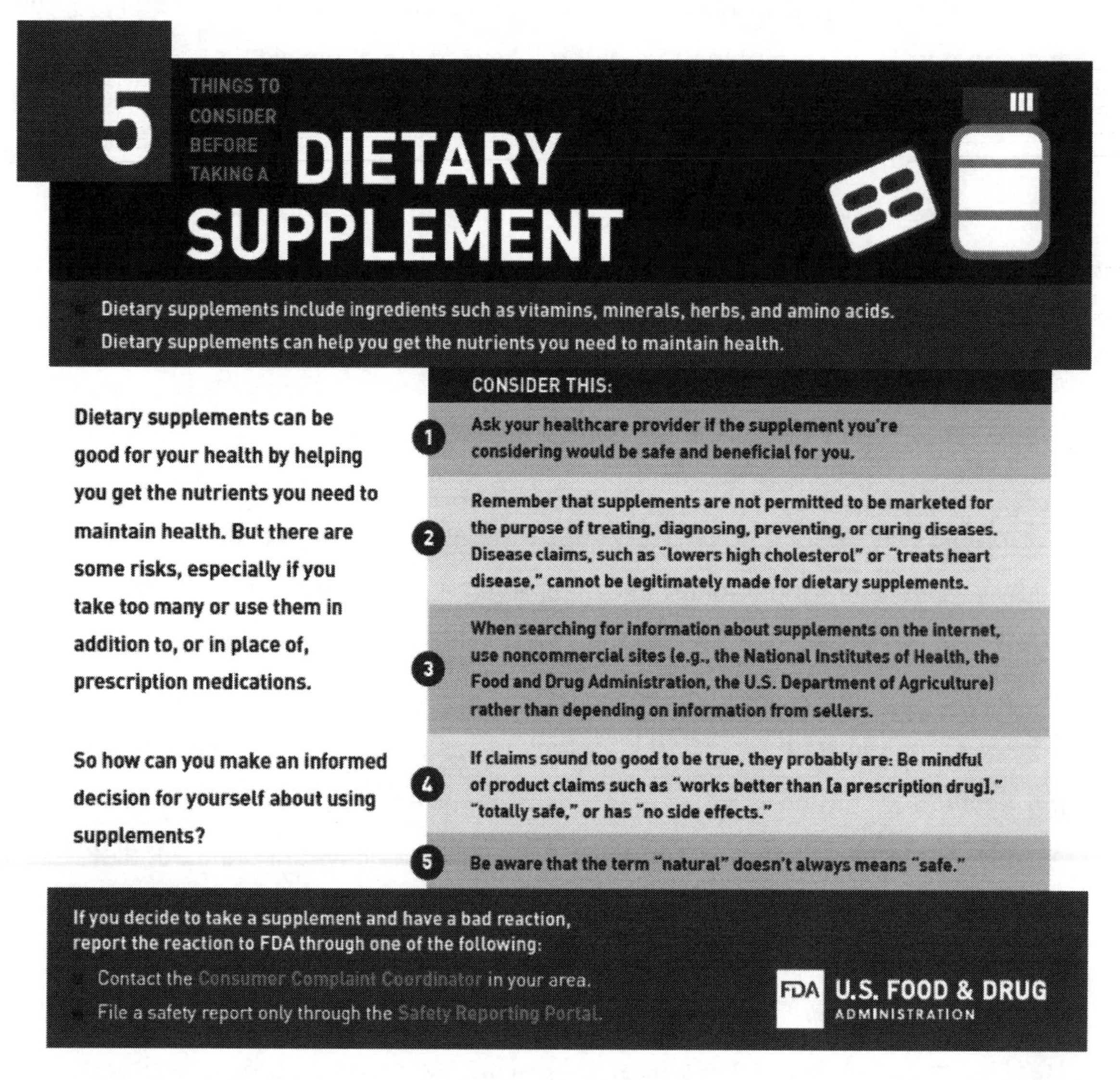

Figure 9. Things to Consider Before Taking a Dietary Supplement

How to Read a Nutrition Facts Label

The Nutrition Facts label can help guide your nutrient-rich food choices. Yet, only 36% of Americans actually pay attention to this information. Reviewing food labels while shopping can help you choose healthier foods and avoid unhealthy ingredients (See next page).

1) START HERE:
- ✓ What is the serving size?
- ✓ How many servings per container?

Nutrition Facts

Serving Size 1 cup (228g)
Servings Per Container 2

- ➢ Be careful because many foods contain more than one serving!
- ➢ If you eat both servings in this food, you get double the calories.

2) CHECK CALORIES:
- ✓ Are the calories high, low, or just right for your needs?

Amount Per Serving

Calories 250 Calories from Fat 110

- ➢ CALORIE GUIDELINES:
  - **Meals:** 300 – 650 kcals
  - **Snacks:** 150 – 350 kcals

3) WHAT TYPE OF FATS ARE IN THIS FOOD?
- ✓ Avoid all *trans* fat.
- ✓ Saturated fat and cholesterol do **not need to be limited** unless you have a medical condition.

	% Daily Value*
Total Fat 12g	18%
Saturated Fat 3g	15%
Trans Fat 3g	
Cholesterol 30mg	10%
Sodium 470mg	20%
Total Carbohydrate 31g	10%

- ➢ % DAILY VALUE:
  - 5% or less is low
  - 20% or more is high
- ➢ Percentages show how much of each nutrient is provided for a 2,000-calorie diet.

4) CHECK IF GETTING ENOUGH OF THESE NUTRIENTS:
- ✓ Goal for Dietary Fiber is 25-40 grams/day.
- ✓ Vitamin A, C, Calcium and Iron are important. Aim to get 100% through a variety of foods

Dietary Fiber 0g	0%
Sugars 5g	
Protein 5g	
Vitamin A	4%
Vitamin C	2%
Calcium	20%
Iron	4%

- ➢ PROTEIN:
  - Protein in your meals and snacks improves satiety and helps you manage your weight. Minimum protein depends on carbohydrates. Aim for no more than a 4:1 carb:protein ratio (i.e., 40g carbs, 10g protein)

5) FOOT NOTES:
- ✓ Describes how much of each nutrient is recommended for a person if eating a 2,000 or 2,500 calorie diet.

* Percent Daily Values are based on a 2,000 calorie diet. Your Daily Values may be higher or lower depending on your calorie needs.

	Calories:	2,000	2,500
Total Fat	Less than	65g	80g
Sat Fat	Less than	20g	25g
Cholesterol	Less than	300mg	300mg
Sodium	Less than	2,400mg	2,400mg
Total Carbohydrate		300g	375g
Dietary Fiber		25g	30g

- ➢ The foot note guides the % Daily Values numbers.
- ➢ However, each person has different needs and these numbers are only guidelines.

Activity #3: Reading a Food Label

Choose a food that you commonly eat and answer the following questions by looking at the food label information (If you do not have the food with you, feel free to look up the information online).

- Name of Product: ________________
- Serving size: ________________
  - Amount of servings per package: ____________
- Total Calories per serving: ________________
  - Total Calories per package: ________________
- Total Fat (g): ________________
  - Percentage of daily value from Fat: ___________
  - Saturated Fat (g): ________________
  - Trans Fat (g): ________________
- Cholesterol (mg): ________________
- Sodium (mg): ________________
- Total Carbohydrates (g): ________________
- Dietary Fiber (g): ________________
- Sugars (g): ________________
- Protein (g): ________________

QUESTIONS:

1) List any claims made on the label (i.e. Fat-Free, Low- Sodium etc.):
2) List the Vitamins and Minerals and their % Daily Values:
3) What was the first ingredient listed in the list of ingredients?
4) List any ingredients from the ingredient list that you wouldn't know where to purchase in a grocery store: (i.e. hydrogenated cottonseed oil)
5) After answering these questions and examining the food label and list of ingredients, would you consider this food a healthy option? Why or why not?

Ingredient Labels: Top Ingredients to Avoid

When reading the ingredient label, watch out for these items because they have negative effects on your health and vitality.

HIGH FRUCTOSE CORN SYRUP OR CORN SYRUP

High fructose corn syrup, also called HFCS, is in so much of our food that it is almost impossible to completely avoid. It may be cheaper to produce and use in products than sugar, but our bodies don't seem to like it very much. It's very hard to digest and convert to fuel, and it can cause inflammation in vital organs and age our skin faster. It also seems to be a big contributing factor when it comes to obesity, so it's wise to ensure it's not in your food.

HYDROGENATED OR PARTIALLY HYDROGENATED OILS

Partially hydrogenated oils are found in thousands of processed foods (breakfast cereals, cookies, chips, deep-fried foods) and are the major source of *trans* fatty acids. *Trans* fats are proven to cause heart disease and contribute to obesity. Consequences of a diet rich in *trans* fats include: increased inflammation, decreased immune function, decreased testosterone, arthritis, cancer, decreased IQ, diabetes, high blood pressure and liver damage. Some foods naturally contain small amounts of *trans* fats, like dairy, where *trans* fats are ok.

ARTIFICIAL FOOD COLORINGS

Artificial colorings may make food look nice, but the effects on our health are controversial. These synthetic substances have no nutritional value and have been linked to cancer, tumors, and allergic reactions. Artificial colors include: FD&C Blue Nos. 1 and 2, FD&C Green No. 3, FD&C Red Nos. 3 and 40, FD&C Yellow Nos. 5 and 6, Orange B, and Citrus Red No. 2 – make sure these are not in your food. Food manufacturers have recognized consumer dislike for artificial food colors and have started to use more natural colorings from fruits and vegetables.

ARTIFICIAL AND IMITATION FLAVORS

Some of the more common artificial flavors include artificial butter, imitation vanilla (vanillin), cherry, banana, raspberry, lemon, and many other flavors. These are synthetically developed and are likely to contain unhealthy contaminants originating from the manufacturing process.

MSG (MONOSODIUM GLUTAMATE)

Monosodium glutamate is a chemical that has been associated with reproductive disorders (it's linked to reduced fertility), migraine headaches, permanent damage to the endocrine system leading to obesity, and other serious disorders. MSG is used in many foods as a taste enhancer. You will rarely see "MSG" on a list of ingredients. It is usually hidden within other common ingredients such as yeast extract, autolyzed vegetable protein or hydrolyzed vegetable protein – all three of which contain MSG and should be avoided.

SODIUM NITRITE/NITRATE

Sodium Nitrite is added to many packaged and deli counter meat products, to add red coloring to meats to make them look fresher and more appetizing. The "sodium" in the name leaves many people thinking it is a form of salt, but Sodium Nitrite is, in fact, a carcinogen (a cancer-causing substance) that has been linked to brain tumors, leukemia and cancers of the digestive tract. Amazingly this is an "accepted" ingredient and you will find no warnings on food labels.

TRACE INGREDIENTS, INCIDENTAL ADDITIVES, AND PROPRIETARY BLENDS

The FDA does not require a breakdown of ingredients in cases where a "company blend" is proprietary, or in cases where a trace ingredient is insignificant to the overall food product. Some ingredients may not be fully disclosed to protect a company's secret formula. If you're trying to avoid a particular ingredient, use caution when you see these generic statements on ingredients labels, because you don't really know what these secret formulas and blends may contain.

Nutrition for a Heathy Body Composition

What is Body Composition?

Body composition is the measure of fat, muscle, and bone in the human body. Assessing body composition is one method to evaluate nutritional status, which is directly related to health. Your body weight does not fully describe the specific composition of your body since this value is made up of fat (both essential fat and storage fat), muscle (protein), bone (minerals), and water. Two people may have the same body weight, but have very different body compositions, in particular the amount of muscle and fat they carry.

Often body composition is measured to assess risk for development of diseases related to lifestyle, especially dietary intake and levels of physical activity. As such, body composition is important to evaluate the current state of an person's body and their risk of future disease.

Two of the commonly most looked at areas of body composition are body fat and body muscle. Of body fat, we have two types: essential fat and storage fat. Essential fat is the minimum amount of fat needed for good health, while storage fat is the fat deposited in adipose tissue (fat cells) that protects our organs and insulates our body. Women have higher amounts of both essential and storage fat, due to fat that makes up their breast tissue and fat needed to support reproduction. As such, women have higher total body fat levels than men.

For body muscle—part of our fat-free tissue—higher amounts of lean muscle is related to lower rates of disease risk. Athletes have more lean tissue than non-athletes because physical activity builds and maintains muscle mass. For ideal health and body composition, physical activity and proper diet is important.

How Do You Measure Body Composition?

There are several ways you can assess your body composition. Some you can do yourself at home, while others require expensive equipment operated by trained technicians. Regardless of the method you use, it's important to measure yourself (or have yourself measured) in the same state each time – meaning the same time of day, the same stage of your menstrual cycle (for women), while you are fasting (no food or water), or after a similar meal, and by the same method type and technician to avoid measurement errors.

Anthropometry

Anthropometric measurements are the most basic method of assessing body composition. These measurements describe body mass, size, shape, and level of fatness. Most of the methods are simple and reliable ways to determine body composition. They include Body Mass Index (BMI), body circumferences, and skinfold thickness.

Body Mass Index (BMI)

BMI uses your height and weight and compares this to a standardized chart to determine if you are underweight, healthy, or overweight. A high BMI can be an indicator of high body fatness. BMI can be used to screen for weight categories that may lead to health problems, but it is not diagnostic of the body fatness or health of an individual. However, BMI appears to be as strongly correlated with various metabolic and disease outcome. In general, BMI is an inexpensive and easy-to-perform method of screening for weight categories.

BODY MASS INDEX	CLASSIFICATION
Less than 18.5	Underweight
18.5 – 24.9	Normal
25 – 29.9	Overweight
30 – 34.9	Mildy Obese
35.0 – 39.9	Moderately Obese
40 or greater	Severely Obese

Source: www.nhlbi.nih.gov

Activity #4: Calculate your BMI

Calculate your BMI, then classify yourself as either underweight, normal weight, overweight, mildly obese, moderately obese, or severely obese. A sample is provided on the next page.

$$BMI = \frac{\text{Weight (kg)}^2}{\text{(Height in meters)}^2} \quad \text{OR} \quad BMI = \frac{703 \times \text{Weight (lb)}}{\text{(Height in inches)}^2}$$

Example: You are a female who weighs 150 lbs and is 5‘5“ (65“) tall.

Calculation for BMI: $[150/ (65)^2] \times 703$ = **24.98 - Normal Weight**

NOW CALCULATE YOUR OWN BMI:

CLASSIFY YOUR CATEGORY:

How Good is BMI as an Indicator of Body Fatness?

The correlation between the BMI and body fatness is fairly strong but even if two people have the same BMI, their level of body fatness may differ.
In general,

- At the same BMI, women tend to have more body fat than men
- At the same BMI, African Americans have less body fat than do whites and asians have more body fat than do whites
- At the same BMI, older people, on average, tend to have more body fat than younger adults
- At the same BMI, athletes have less body fat than do non-athletes

The accuracy of BMI as an indicator of body fatness also appears to be higher in persons with higher levels of BMI and body fatness. While, a person with a very high BMI is very likely to have high body fat, a relatively high BMI can be the result of either high body fat or high lean body mass (muscle and bone). A trained healthcare provider should perform appropriate health assessments in order to evaluate an individual's health status and risks.

Body Circumferences

Circumferenes, also called girths, includes measuring the circumference of different parts of the body such as the waist (abdomen, the hips, the neck, and the upper and lower extremeties. The most common measurement sites are the waist and hips.

With regards to the abdomen (waist), obesity is commonly associated with increased amounts of intra-abdominal fat (fat around the organs in the middle of the body). People with a big abdomen usually have a large amount of both intra-abdominal and subcutaneous (under the skin) fat, which puts them at greater risk of disease. Measurement of waist circumference is a simple way to determine if a person has too much central abdominal body fat. A waist circumference of 40 inches or more in men, or 35 inches or more in women, is associated with health problems, such as Type 2 diabetes, heart disease, and high blood pressure.

Waist circumference is often compared to hip circumference (known as the waist-to-hip ratio; WHR). WHR is a measurement tool that compares the proportion of fat stored on your waist to the fat on your hips/buttocks. Weight concentrated around the middle is often referred to as an "apple" shape; whereas weight concentrated around the hips is referred to as a "pear" shape.

Activity #5: Calculate your WHR

Using the three easy steps below, measure your Waist-Hip Ratio (WHR). Then classify yourself as "at-risk" or "reduced-risk"

Standard ratios for WHR that are considered reduced risk of diseases:

- Women: Less than 0.80
- Men: Less than 0.95

HOW TO CALCULATE:

1. Using a flexible tape measure, measure your waist - just under your lowest rib and at the top of your hip bone
2. Bring the tape measure all the way around your body, level with your belly button to measure your hips – this should be at the widest portion of your buttocks.
3. Divide waist measurement by hip measurement to get the ratio.

CLASSIFY YOUR WHR:

Skinfold Thickness

A skinfold thickness measurement provides an estimated size of the subcutaneous fat deposit, which is the fat under the skin. We know that in most people, approximately half of the body's fat is stored under the skin. By estimating the thickness of this area, researchers are able to obtain an estimation of the total body fat using special calculations. The goal of this method is to provide an assessment of body fatness, which is a better method than BMI.

In order to obtain this measurement, you need to go to a trained technician who will use a tool called skin fold calipers. It's very easy to have inaccuracies in this method because of poor measurer technique. Proper technique involves pinching the skin between the index finger and thumb and measuring specific sites on the body. According to the National Health and Nutrition Examination Survey (NHANES), these measures should be on the right side of the body. When this method is performed by a skilled technician, it can estimate body fatness with an error of 3-4%. This means that if your skinfold shows you have 20% body fat, your actual value could be as low as 16% or as high as 24%.

Other Measurements of Body Composition

Three more advanced measurements of body composition include Underwater Weighing, Dual-Energy X-ray Absorptiometery (DEXA), and Bod Pod. These methods all require the use of specialized equipement and a trained technician. In underwater weighing, a person is submerged underwater, and the amount of water that his or her body dispaces is converted to a measure of body density and then an estimate of body fat. This method is considered quite accurate when performed correctly. In DEXA, this technology is based on using very low-level x-rays to distinguish between bone, muscle and fat. In involves lying on a specialized table while x-rays are passed through the body and the image is displayed on a screen.

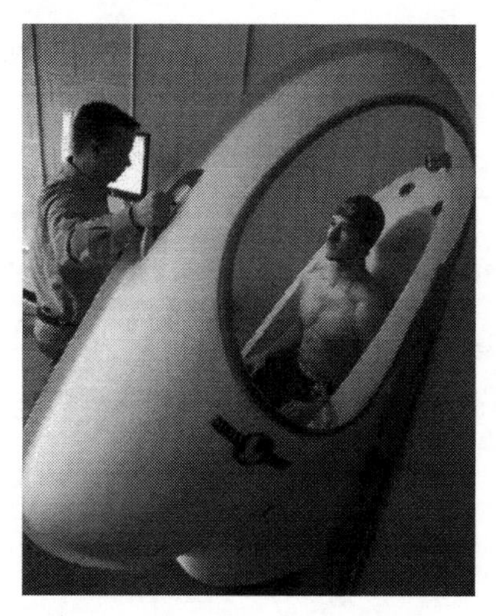

Figure 10. BOD POD at CCSU

Here at CCSU, we have the BOD POD (Figure 10), which uses air displacment to estimate body composition. This machine is a large, egg-shaped chamber, in which a person is enclosed. If you take Exercise Science classes at CCSU, you will learn more about this machine and can have your body composition tested. Testing services for a fee are also available through the Department of Physical Education and Human Performance.

What is a Healthy Body Composition?

A healthy body composition is usually determined by the amount of body fatness a person has – both essential and storage fat. Essential body fat is present in the nerve tissues, bone marrow, and organs (all membranes), and we cannot lose this fat without compromising physiological function. Storage fat, on the other hand, represents an energy reserve that accumulates when excess energy is ingested and decreases when more energy is expended than consumed. Essential body fat is approximately 3-5% of body mass for men and 8-12% of body mass for women. Women are believed to have more essential body fat than men because of childbearing and hormonal functions. In general, the total body fat percentage (essential plus storage fat) is between 12% and 15% for young men and between 25% and 28% for young women; younger women have a larger range of body fat than this (less and more for both genders).

How Does Your Diet Influence Your Body Composition?

You may have heard the saying: "*You can't out-exercise a bad diet.*"

What this essentially means is that exercise will not overcome the negative effects on your health and body composition of an unhealthy diet (or a diet too high in calories for your needs). As such, the combination of regular physical activity paired with a diet that is adequate, moderate, balanced, nutrient dense, and varied will promote the most ideal body composition for you.

Keep in mind, many factors influence body composition beyond diet and exercise:

- ✓ Genetics – you will likely look like your parents when you are their age
- ✓ Hormones – certain hormones cause your body to gain muscle or store fat
- ✓ Certain prescription medications, such as anxiety medications, anti-depressants, and anti-inflammtory drugs
- ✓ Age and socioeconomic factors – you're more likely to gain body fat when you are older or have had children, people who have less money for nutritious food may have to survive off high calorie junk foods.

Overall, a healthy body composition is one that is right for you. You are unique and only meant to look a certain way. There are limits to the way you can change your body and you should never risk your health to reduce your body fat to dangerously low levels. Body image and body acceptance can occur in all body types, and it's most important to love your body the way you were made and always strive to keep it healthy and strong versus lean and sick. Make sure you focus on wholesome foods and eat to support physical activity and proper mental function. Never starve yourself – food is good and should be eaten. Just be mindful of your portion sizes and how many calories you're eating each day. If you find yourself struggling to maintain an ideal body weight or body fat percentage, look closely at your diet and your participation in physical activity.

Chapter Summary

- ✓ A healthy diet is one that is adequate, moderate, balanced, nutrient dense, and varied. An unhealthy diet is any consistent food intake that promotes unnecessary weight/body fat gain, causes gut dysfunction, leads to anxiety or poor sleep, causes allergies, intolerances and/or illnesses, makes it hard to focus, feel well, and have positive mental clarity.
- ✓ Vegetarians do not eat meat, fish, and poultry. Some vegetarians eat eggs and/or dairy. Vegans are vegetarians who abstain from eating or using all animal products, including milk, cheese, other dairy items, eggs, honey, wool, silk, or leather.
- ✓ Nutrients are classified into two categories. The major essential nutrients include carbohydrates, proteins, fats, and water, which are required in large amounts, and, other than water, provide our body with energy. The minor nutrients are required in lesser amounts and include vitamins and minerals and other nutrients that help our body make energy and prevent diseases.
- ✓ When reading a food label there are some ingredients you should look out for which include, high fructose corn syrup, hydrogenated, and partially hydrogenated oils, artificial food colorings, artificial and imitation flavors, MSG, sodium nitrite/nitrate, trace ingredients, incidental additives, and proprietary blends.
- ✓ Body Mass Index (BMI) can help establish if a person is at risk for health problems. BMI uses your height and weight and compares this to a standardized chart to determine if you are underweight, healthy, or overweight. A high BMI can be an indicator of high body fatness.
- ✓ Waist-Hip Ratio (WHR) is another tool that can determine if a person is at risk for health problems. WHR compares the proportion of fat stored on your waist to the fat on your hips/buttocks. Weight concentrated around the middle is often referred to as an "apple" shape; whereas weight concentrated around the hips is referred to as a "pear" shape.

- ✓ A healthy body composition is usually determined by percent of body fat the individual has. Essential body fat is needed for physiological function. Storage fat represents an energy reserve that accumulates when excess energy is ingested.

Chapter Review Questions

1) What is the definition of nutrition and what are five components of a healthy diet?
2) Describe five ways you can get the recommended amounts of fruits and vegetables in your diet each day? What are the current recommendations for fruits and vegetable intake?
3) What is the difference between a vegetarian and vegan diet?
4) What are two food groups that are rich in dietary fiber? How would you incorporate these foods into your daily food intake?
5) Why do we eat dietary protein? Does it provide much usable energy for everyday functions?
6) Why are *trans* fats so bad for our health?
7) What are four food/beverage sources of water for our body?
8) What are reasons why you would take a dietary supplement?
9) What are the two types of body fat we have? Describe them.
10) Calculate your waist-hip ratio (WHR). What is it? Is it considered healthy?
11) Describe what you learned about having a healthy body composition. What is a healthy body composition?

References

Center for Disease Control and Prevention. (CDC, 2017) *About Adult BMI* from **www.cdc.gov/healthyweight/assessing/bmi/adult_bmi/index.html**

National Institutes of Health (NIH, n.d.) Dietary Supplements Fact Sheets from: **https://ods.od.nih.gov/factsheets/list-all/**

Thompson, J. & Manore, M. (2017). *Nutrition: An applied approach*, 5th edition. New York, NY: Pearson.

United States Department of Agriculture (USDA, n.d.) *Choose My Plate* from: **www.choosemyplate.gov**

Chapter 4

Mental Health Wellness

By Cassandra Forsythe York, PhD, RD

Chapter Objectives

After reading this chapter, students should be able to:

- ✓ Understand mental health as an important element of emotional, psychological, and social well-being;
- ✓ Understand the factors that contribute to disruptions in mental well-being;
- ✓ Compare mental disorder as opposed to mental illness;
- ✓ Understand anxiety disorders, as well as treatments of anxiety disorders;
- ✓ Understand the impacts and effects among college students of eating disorders and traumatic events, such as military combat, assault, an accident or a natural disaster; and
- ✓ Understand relationships among attempts at suicide, alcohol, and addiction with respect mental illnesses.

Mental Health Wellness

"The best view comes after the hardest climb" – Unknown

What is Mental Health?

Mental health is an important topic that encompasses our emotional, psychological and social well-being. A positive sense of well-being enables a person to function normally in society and meet the demands of everyday life. It also helps determine how you handle stress and relate to others. Being emotionally well means feeling positive about yourself and your environment. However, every person from time to time experiences sadness, or uncertainty – that is normal. It's when these negative emotions overcome your positive emotions that your well-being will suffer.

Everybody experiences many different emotions: happy, sad, angry, excited, embarrassed, anxious, hurt, scared, in love. The range of our emotions is so great that we even use emojis on our smart phones to digitally express how we are feeling to others (Figure 1).

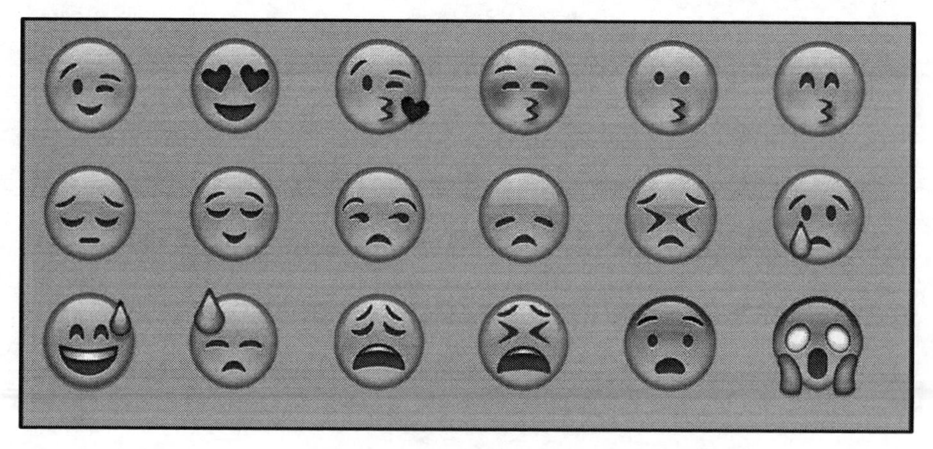

Figure 1. Emojis to express emotions

These emotions make up our mental health, which, just like emojis, should vary depending on the situation. If you find yourself expressing only negative or sad emotions to others, you may have a mental health disorder or illness.

Mental Health Disorders and Illnesses

Over the course of your life, if you experience mental health problems, your thinking, mood, and behavior could be affected. Many factors contribute to disruptions in your mental well-being, including:

- ✓ Biological factors, such as genes or brain chemistry
- ✓ Life experiences, such as trauma or abuse
- ✓ Family history of mental health problems

When you have a significant disruption in your mental well-being, you may develop a mental health disorder, better known as a mental illness.

A **MENTAL DISORDER** is considered any disturbance or derangement in your mental health, while a **MENTAL ILLNESS** refers to a wide range of mental health conditions that affect your mood, thinking and behavior. Examples of mental illnesses include depression, anxiety disorders, eating disorders and addictive behaviors.

Any of these mental health conditions are not the result of one event or factor. As stated, many factors contribute to the well-being of your mental health, such that they may develop slowly over time until they get to the point where you need to take action.

Warning signs of a significant mental health disturbance include:

- ✓ Eating or sleeping too much or too little
- ✓ Pulling away from people and usual activities
- ✓ Having low or no energy
- ✓ Feeling numb or like nothing matters
- ✓ Having unexplained aches and pains
- ✓ Feeling helpless or hopeless
- ✓ Smoking, drinking, or using drugs more than usual
- ✓ Feeling unusually forgetful, on edge, angry, upset, worried, or scared
- ✓ Yelling or fighting with family and friends

- ✓ Experiencing severe mood swings that cause problems in relationships
- ✓ Having persistent thoughts and memories you can't get out of your head
- ✓ Thinking of harming yourself or others
- ✓ Inability to perform daily tasks like getting to work or school

Mental illnesses are more common than you would expect. The following infographic from the National Alliance on Mental Illness outlines statistics and facts on mental health in America (Figure 2).

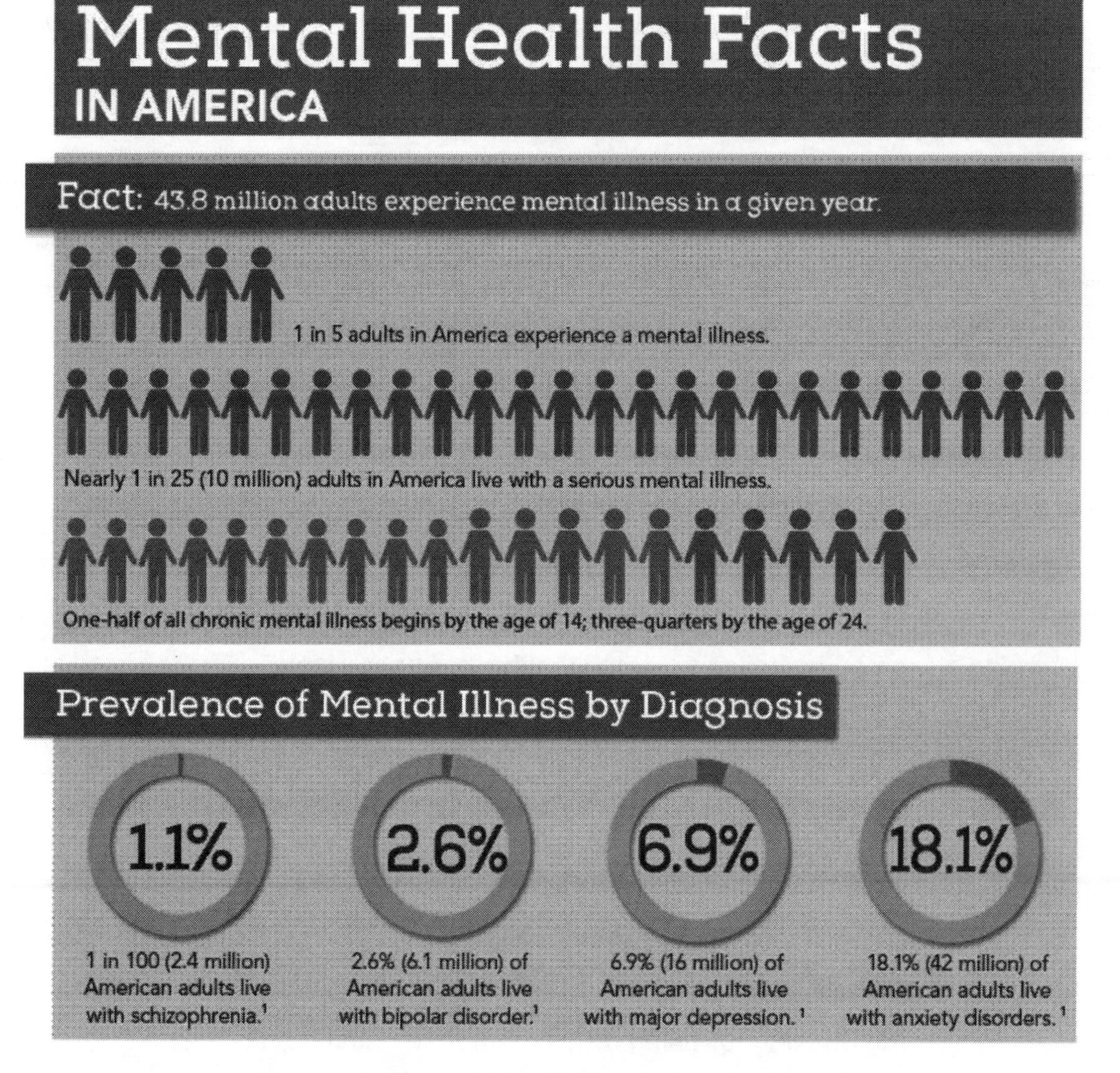

Figure 2. Mental Health Statistics in America

Source: NAMI, www.nami.org

CCSU Student Wellness Services Contact Information

APPOINTMENT LINE (860) 832-1926

General Inquiries (860) 832-1925

Wellness Education- Educational Programming (860) 832- 1948

Monday- Friday 8:00am-5:00 pm

Marcus White Annex next to Student Technology

If you are experiencing a mental health problem, you are not alone because 1 in 5 adults experience a mental health condition every year. Half of mental health conditions begin by age 14, and 75% of mental health conditions develop by age 24. So, for college students, you may just start seeing a change in your mental well-being, which may develop into a more serious condition. If you are struggling, please make an appointment at Student Wellness Services at CCSU.

The following are the most common mental health illnesses that college students face today.

Depressive Disorder

Depressive disorder, frequently referred to simply as depression, is more than just feeling sad or going through a rough patch. It's a serious mental health condition that requires understanding and medical care. Some will only experience one depressive episode in a lifetime, but for most, depressive disorder recurs. Without treatment, episodes may last a few months to several years.

An estimated 16 million American adults—almost 7% of the population—had at least one major depressive episode in the past year. People of all ages and all racial, ethnic and socioeconomic backgrounds experience depression, but it does affect some groups more than others. Left untreated, depression can be devastating for those who have it, and their families. Fortunately, with early detection, diagnosis and a treatment plan consisting of medication, psychotherapy and healthy lifestyle choices, many people can and do get better.

Depression can present different symptoms, depending on the person. But for most people, depressive disorder changes how they function day-to-day, and typically for more than two weeks. Common symptoms of depression are presented in the image below (Figure 3). To be diagnosed with depressive disorder, a person must have experienced a depressive episode lasting longer than two weeks.

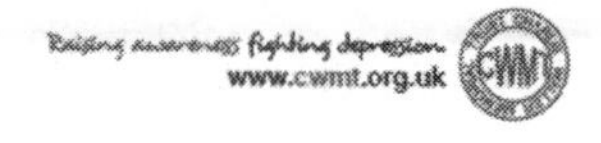

Figure 3. Warning Signs of Depression

Depression does not have a single cause. It can be triggered by a life crisis, physical illness or something else—but it can also occur spontaneously. Scientists believe several factors can contribute to depression:

- ✓ **TRAUMA.** When people experience trauma at an early age, it can cause long-term changes in how their brains respond to fear and stress. These changes may lead to depression.
- ✓ **GENETICS.** Mood disorders, such as depression, tend to run in families.
- ✓ **LIFE CIRCUMSTANCES.** The transition to college is a huge change that can trigger depression in many people. Relationship changes, financial standing and where a person lives influence also whether a person develops depression.
- ✓ **BRAIN CHANGES.** Imaging studies have shown that the frontal lobe of the brain becomes less active when a person is depressed. Depression is also associated with changes in how the pituitary gland and hypothalamus respond to hormone stimulation.
- ✓ **OTHER MEDICAL CONDITIONS.** People who have a history of sleep disturbances, medical illness, chronic pain, anxiety and attention-deficit hyperactivity disorder (ADHD) are more likely to develop depression. Some medical syndromes (like hypothyroidism) can mimic depressive disorder. Some medications can also cause symptoms of depression.
- ✓ **DRUG AND ALCOHOL ABUSE.** Approximately 30% of people with substance abuse problems also have depression. This requires coordinated treatment for both conditions, as alcohol can worsen symptoms.

Treatments for Depression

Although depressive disorder can be devastating, confusing and maybe even embarrassing, it often responds very well to treatment. The key is to get a specific evaluation and treatment plan for your unique condition which requires meeting with a medical doctor or psychiatrist. These professionals can rule out any confounding medical problems and other possible causes that are contributing to your symptoms.

If you are contemplating suicide, please let someone know so they can check on you and help keep you safe. The key is to not be ashamed to seek out help and recognize that treatment will assist in your recovery to ideal well-being – struggling with depression is not your fault, and you do not have to suffer from it.

Your path to wellness may include any or a combination of the following:

- ✓ **Psychotherapy** (counseling) including cognitive behavioral therapy, family-focused therapy and interpersonal therapy.
- ✓ **Medications** including antidepressants, mood stabilizers and antipsychotic medications. Your doctor will work with you to find the medication that is best for you.
- ✓ **Brain stimulation therapies** can be tried if psychotherapy and/or medication are not effective. These include electroconvulsive therapy (ECT) for depressive disorder with psychosis or repetitive transcranial magnetic stimulation (rTMS) for severe depression.
- ✓ **Light therapy**, which uses a light box to expose a person to full spectrum light to regulate the hormone melatonin.
- ✓ **Alternative approaches** including acupuncture, meditation, faith and nutrition can be part of a comprehensive treatment plan.
- ✓ **Exercise** can help with prevention and mild-to-moderate symptoms.

Anxiety Disorders

Experiencing anxiety when you take an exam or give a presentation in front of a class is normal. However, when feelings of intense fear and distress are overwhelming and prevent you from doing everyday things, an anxiety disorder may be the cause. Most people develop symptoms of anxiety disorders before age 21, and women are 60% more likely to be diagnosed with an anxiety disorder than men.

Anxiety disorders are a group of related conditions, and each with unique symptoms. However, all anxiety disorders have one thing in common: persistent, excessive fear or worry in situations that are not threatening. Other emotional and physical symptoms include:

- ✓ Feelings of apprehension or dread
- ✓ Sweating, tremors or twitches
- ✓ Upset stomach, frequent urination or diarrhea

The most common anxiety disorders include:

- ✓ **PANIC DISORDER** which is characterized by panic attacks—sudden feelings of terror—sometimes striking repeatedly and without warning. A panic attack sometimes is mistaken for a heart attack because it causes powerful, physical symptoms including chest pain, heart palpitations, dizziness, shortness of breath and stomach upset.
- ✓ **PHOBIAS** which are reactions of strong, irrational fear of certain places, events or objects. Most people with specific phobias have several triggers. To avoid panicking, someone with specific phobias will work hard to avoid their triggers. Depending on the type and number of triggers, this fear and the attempt to control it can seem to take over a person's life.
- ✓ **GENERALIZED ANXIETY DISORDER** that produces chronic, exaggerated worrying about everyday life. This can consume hours each day, making it hard to concentrate or finish routine daily tasks.
- ✓ **SOCIAL ANXIETY DISORDER** which leads to intense fear, often driven by irrational worries about social humiliation – "saying something stupid," or "not knowing what to say." Someone with social anxiety disorder may not take part in conversations, contribute to class discussions, or offer their ideas, and may become isolated. Panic attack symptoms are a common reaction.

Treatments for Anxiety Disorders

Treatment for anxiety disorders are very similar to the treatment for depression and should first and foremost start with psychotherapy (meeting with a mental health professional) complimented with healthy lifestyle approaches such as stress and relaxation techniques, better nutrition (See Chapter 3) and regular, enjoyable physical activity. If these methods are not enough, medications may be prescribed, which can be very useful for people who are affected deeply by any of these anxiety disorders.

The Anxiety and Depression Association of America (ADAA; www.adaa.org) has several resources online on topics for treatments of anxiety and depression. One effective treatment to help those struggling with anxiety and depression, along with other disorders, is called Cognitive Behavior Therapy (CBT). The following infographic on the next page from the ADAA explains what CBT is and how it works (Figure 4).

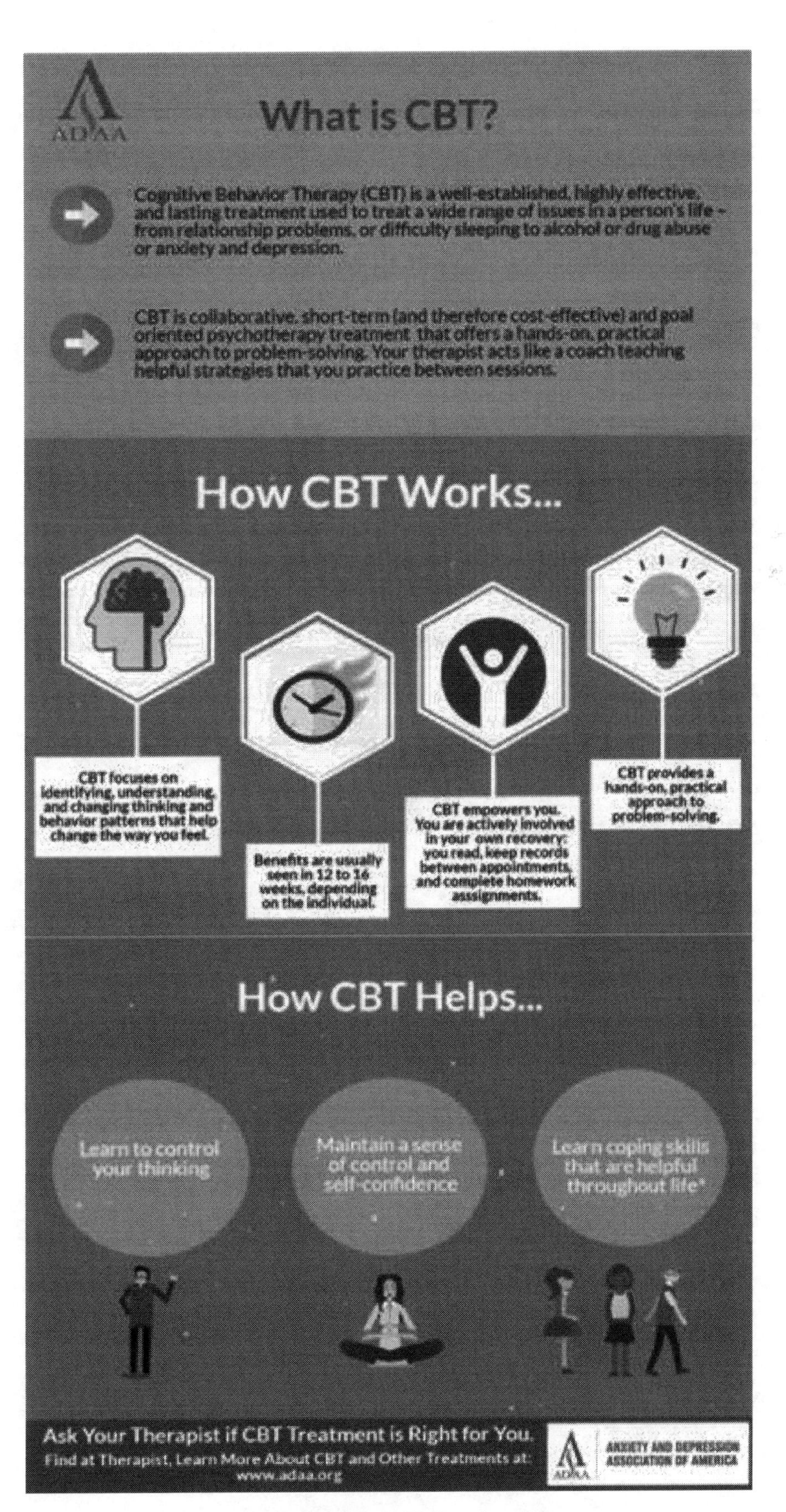

Figure 4. Cognitive Behavior Therapy

After meeting with a therapist/specialist, and engaging in Cognitive Behavior Therapy, you may want to consider the following complimentary therapies to help you deal with depression and anxiety:

- ✓ **STRESS AND RELAXATION TECHNIQUES**
  - Relaxation techniques such as breathing drills and imagery may produce modest short-term reduction of anxiety in people with ongoing health problems.
- ✓ **MEDITATION**
  - Moderate evidence suggests that meditation is useful for symptoms of anxiety and depression in adults.
- ✓ **YOGA**
  - Yoga, which combines physical postures, breathing exercises, meditation, and a distinct philosophy, is one of the top ten practices of CAM (complementary and alternative medicine). It may also help alleviate anxiety and depression.
- ✓ **ACUPUNCTURE**
  - Evidence for use of acupuncture — the Chinese practice of inserting needles into the body at specific points to manipulates the body's flow of energy — to treat anxiety disorders is becoming stronger.

Activity #1: Anxiety Assessment

BECK'S ANXIETY INVENTORY – *See online for full questionnaire*

Below is an example list of common symptoms of anxiety.

Indicate how much you have been bothered by that symptom during the past month, including today.

	Not at all	Mildly but it didn't bother me much	Moderately- it wasn't pleasant at times	Severely- it bothered me a lot
Numbness or tingling				
Feeling hot				
Wobbliness in legs				
Unable to Relax				
Fear of worst happening				

Activity #2: Depression Assessment

BECK'S DEPRESSION INVENTORY – *See online for full questionnaire*

This depression inventory can be self-scored. The scoring scale is at the end of the questionnaire. The following are example questions.

A:
0). I do not feel sad.
1). I feel sad
2). I am sad all the time and I can't snap out of it.
3). I am so sad and unhappy that I can't stand it.

B:
0). I am not particularly discouraged about the future.
1). I feel discouraged about the future.
2). I feel I have nothing to look forward to.
3). I feel the future is hopeless and that things cannot improve.

C:
0). I do not feel like a failure.
1). I feel I have failed more than the average person.
2). As I look back on my life, all I can see is a lot of failures.
3). I feel I am a complete failure as a person.

Eating Disorders

When you become so preoccupied with food and your body weight that you find it harder and harder to focus on other aspects of your life, it may be an early sign of an eating disorder. The National Institute of Mental Health estimates that 25 percent of all college students struggle with an eating disorder (ED) and both females and males are affected. The figure below outlines the seriousness of eating disorders, specifically that eating disorders are the #1 killer of people who struggle with mental health illnesses (Figure 5).

Warning Signs: Eating Disorders

People with eating disorders risk premature death due to medical complications.

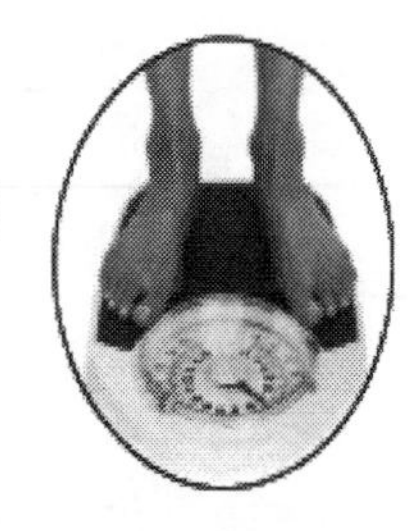

- Low self esteem and body image
- Dramatic weight loss
- Preoccupation with weight, food facts, meal rituals
- Routine bathroom trips immediately after eating
- Binging on and hoarding large amounts of food
- Increased use of laxatives, diuretics or diet pills
- Compulsive exercising
- Withdrawn from friends and activities

Source: National Eating Disorders Association

Figure 5. Warning Signs of ED

College students are greatly affected by eating disorders because this is the time when they struggle with identity issues, one of the core issues involved with this disorder. College is a time when previous eating disorders may worse, or they can develop for the first time. Without treatment, eating disorders can take over a person's life and lead to serious, potentially fatal medical complications. As such, recognizing the warning signs of eating disorders is incredibly important.

Eating disorders are more than just one type. They are a group of related conditions that involve extreme food and body weight issues; however, each has unique symptoms that separate it from the others.

ANOREXIA NERVOSA. A person with anorexia will deny themselves food to the point of self-starvation as he or she obsesses about weight loss. With anorexia, a person will deny hunger and refuse to eat, practice binge eating and purging behaviors or exercise to the point of exhaustion as she attempts to limit, eliminate or "burn" calories.

The emotional symptoms of anorexia include irritability, social withdrawal, lack of mood or emotion, not able to understand the seriousness of the situation, fear of eating in public and obsessions with food and exercise. Often food rituals are developed or whole categories of food are eliminated from the diet, out of fear of being "fat".

Anorexia can take a heavy physical toll. Very low food intake and inadequate nutrition causes a person to become very thin. The body is forced to slow down to conserve energy causing irregularities or loss of menstruation, constipation and abdominal pain, irregular heart rhythms, low blood pressure, dehydration and trouble sleeping. Some people with anorexia might also use binge eating and purge behaviors, while others only restrict eating.

BULIMIA NERVOSA. Someone living with bulimia will feel out of control when binging on very large amounts of food during short periods of time, and then desperately try to rid himself of the extra calories using forced vomiting, abusing laxatives or excessive exercise. This becomes a repeating cycle that controls many aspects of the person's life and has a very negative effect both emotionally and physically. People living with bulimia are usually normal weight or even a bit overweight.

The emotional symptoms of bulimia include low self-esteem overly linked to body image, feelings of being out of control, feeling guilty or shameful about eating and withdrawal from friends and family.

Like anorexia, bulimia will inflict physical damage. The binging and purging can severely harm the parts of the body involved in eating and digesting food, teeth are damaged by frequent vomiting, and acid reflux is common. Excessive purging can cause dehydration that effect the body's electrolytes and leads to cardiac arrhythmias, heart failure and even death.

BINGE EATING DISORDER (BED). A person with BED losses control over his eating and eats a very large amount of food in a short period of time. He may also eat large amounts of food even when he isn't hungry or after he is uncomfortably full. This causes him to feel embarrassed, disgusted, depressed or guilty about his behavior. A person with BED, after an episode of binge eating, does not attempt to purge or exercise excessively like someone living with anorexia or bulimia would. A person with binge eating disorder may be normal weight, overweight or obese.

Symptoms of eating disorders must meet the criteria in the Diagnostic and Statistical Manual of Mental Disorders (DSM) to warrant a diagnosis. Each eating disorder has its own diagnostic criteria that a mental health professional will use to determine which disorder is involved. It is not necessary to have all the criteria for a disorder to benefit from working with a mental health professional on food and eating issues.

Treatments for Eating Disorders

Often a person with an eating disorder will have symptoms of another mental health condition that requires treatment. Whenever possible, it is best to identified and address all conditions at the same time. This gives a person comprehensive treatment support that helps insure a lasting recovery.

Eating disorders are managed using a variety of techniques. Treatments will vary depending on the type of disorder but will generally include the following.

- ✓ Psychotherapy, such as talk therapy or behavioral therapy.
- ✓ Medicine, such as antidepressants and anti-anxiety drugs. Many people living with an eating disorder often have a co-occurring illness like depression or anxiety, and while there is no medication available to treat eating disorders themselves, many patients find that these medicines help with underlying issues.
- ✓ Nutritional counseling and weight restoration monitoring are also crucial.

Activity #3: Learn more about Eating Disorders

Visit the National Eating Disorders Association (NEDA) at **www.nationaleatingdisorders.org** to learn more about eating disorders and to take online quizzes to see if you are struggling with one. NEDA is the leading non-profit in the field of eating disorders. It supports individuals and families and serves as a catalyst for prevention, cures and access to quality care.

Post-Traumatic Stress Disorder (PTSD)

Traumatic events, such as military combat, assault, an accident or a natural disaster, can have long-lasting negative effects. Sometimes our biological responses and instincts, which can be life-saving during a crisis, leave people with ongoing psychological symptoms because they are not integrated into consciousness.

PTSD affects 3.5% of the U.S. adult population—about 7.7 million Americans—but women are more likely to develop the condition than men. About 37% of those cases are classified as severe. While PTSD can occur at any age, the average age of onset is in a person's early 20s, and many college students, especially those who have served our country oversees, are affected.

Most people who go through a traumatic event have some symptoms at the beginning. Yet only some will develop PTSD. It isn't clear why some people develop PTSD and others don't. How likely you are to get PTSD depends on many things. These include:

- ✓ How intense the trauma was or how long it lasted
- ✓ If you lost someone you were close to or were hurt
- ✓ How close you were to the event
- ✓ How strong your reaction was
- ✓ How much you felt in control of events
- ✓ How much help and support you got after the event

Many people who develop PTSD get better at some time. But about 1 out of 3 people with PTSD may continue to have some symptoms. Even if you continue to have symptoms, treatment can help you cope. Your symptoms don't have to interfere with your everyday activities, work, and relationships

The symptoms of PTSD fall into the following categories.

- ✓ **INTRUSIVE MEMORIES,** which can include flashbacks of reliving the moment of trauma, bad dreams and scary thoughts.
- ✓ **AVOIDANCE,** which can include staying away from certain places or objects that are reminders of the traumatic event. A person may also feel numb, guilty, worried or depressed or having trouble remembering the traumatic event.
- ✓ **DISSOCIATION,** which can include out-of-body experiences or feeling that the world is "not real" (derealization).
- ✓ **HYPERVIGILANCE,** which can include being startled very easily, feeling tense, trouble sleeping or outbursts of anger.

Symptoms of PTSD usually begin within 3 months after a traumatic event, but occasionally emerge years afterward. Symptoms must last more than a month to be considered PTSD. PTSD is often accompanied by depression, substance abuse or another anxiety disorder.

PTSD Treatment

PTSD is treated and managed in several ways.

- ✓ Medications, including mood stabilizers, antipsychotic medications and antidepressants.
- ✓ Psychotherapy, such as cognitive behavioral therapy or group therapy.
- ✓ Self-management strategies, such as "self-soothing". Many therapy techniques, including mindfulness, are helpful to ground a person and bring her back to reality after a dissociative episode or a flashback.
- ✓ Service animals, especially dogs, can help soothe some of the symptoms of PTSD.

Veteran College Student Creating Awareness of PTSD

Bryan Adam's recently presented at CCSU: "My War on PTSD", which recounts his military service as a sniper in Iraq, being wounded in Tikrit, his physical recovery, and his struggle with mental health issues once he returned to civilian life. He candidly discussed his PTSD and anxiety disorder, alcohol abuse and depression, and his continuing care.

His struggles began in 2008 when he was shot during an ambush while on patrol. Bryan came back to the U.S. to pursue his college degree as recipient of a Purple Heart, but nothing could prepare him for how rough the transition would be to campus life and his struggles with post-traumatic stress disorder (PTSD). Today, Bryan shares his moving story of trauma, stigma, and alcohol abuse with active military, veterans, and civilians alike to reinforce the importance of seeking help. A tireless advocate for veterans' rights, Bryan seeks to empower others, and when they cannot speak up for themselves, he hopes that by sharing his story he can speak up for them.

Bryan graduated from Rutgers University with a bachelor's degree in marketing and an impressive resume of work with Active Minds, Iraq and Afghanistan Veterans of America (IAVA), and Student Veterans of America (SVA). Bryan is currently the Veteran Services Coordinator in the Rutgers University Office of Veteran and Military Programs and Services. In that capacity, Bryan is the main point-of-contact for veteran, military, and eligible family members in navigating services within Rutgers University, as well as prospective students. To learn more about Bryan and his work please visit **www.activeminds.org**.

CCSU Counselling and Wellness Center

If you have been diagnosed with PTSD or have personal concerns before or after reviewing this information, please call the CCSU Counselling and Wellness Center at (860) 832-1945 to set up an appointment with one of their counselors. The counselors are here to offer a listening ear, and will not judge, discriminate against, or minimize your concerns.

Suicide Among College Students

Attempts at suicide and death by suicide are most common in college students who struggle with mental illnesses. Depression is cited as a factor, as well as anxiety. Suicide rates among college students have increased by 200 percent since the 1950s, and today, suicide is one of the leading causes of death among college and university students in the United States. Many colleges and universities have mental health facilities, but students may feel uncomfortable about asking for help.

Consider these statistics:

- ✓ There are more than 1,000 suicides on college campuses each year – That's 2-3 deaths by suicide every day
- ✓ More than half of college students have had suicidal thoughts, and 1 in 10 students seriously consider attempting suicide
- ✓ Most importantly: 80-90% of college students who die by suicide were not receiving help from college counseling centers

Suicide attempts and death by suicide are most common in college students who:

- ✓ Are depressed
- ✓ Are either under the influence of substances, or have a substance use problem
- ✓ Have made a previous attempt
- ✓ Have a family history of a mood disorder such as depression or bipolar disorder
- ✓ Are struggling with a history of trauma

It's also recognized that students often tell others when they're emotionally struggling, and that teachers, peers and resident assistants are more adept at recognizing emotional distress among struggling students.

Nevertheless, suicidal students often feel helpless, hopeless, and trapped. Some of these students resist seeking help because they're ashamed. They might fear a "black mark" on their record or being judged by others. Even if they don't have these concerns, they often don't know what services are available.

If you suspect a friend or loved one may be struggling with suicidal thoughts, look for these warning signs in the image below (Figure 6) and let them know you are there for them if they need to talk to someone.

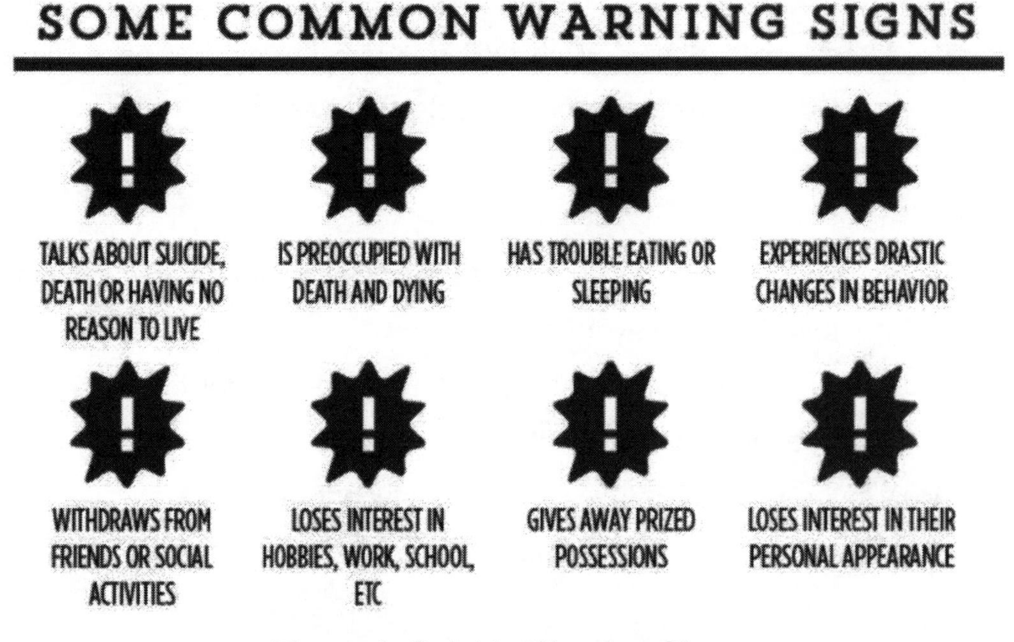

Figure 6. Suicide Warning Signs

If you are struggling emotionally and considering suicide, first think about why ending your life is the answer to your pain. Your loss to this world will leave behind a wake of others who will struggle just as much due to your departure. Suicide also has economic costs for individuals, families, communities, states, and the nation as a whole. These include medical costs for family and friends left behind, lost income for families, and lost productivity for anyone who knew you.

Remember that you won't always feel this way. Depression, anxiety, addiction, sadness, grief, your burning desire to bring yourself harm — none of these things are static states of being. Like all emotions, they are temporary. You will laugh again, you will smile. You will experience more joyful events in life and meet new people who will bring you new experiences and memories. Do your best to hang in there despite the pain you are suffering with right now. And please seek out help from a professional who can give you the support you need. If you can't immediately connect with a professional, call the National Suicide Prevention Lifeline. You are not alone. There is help.

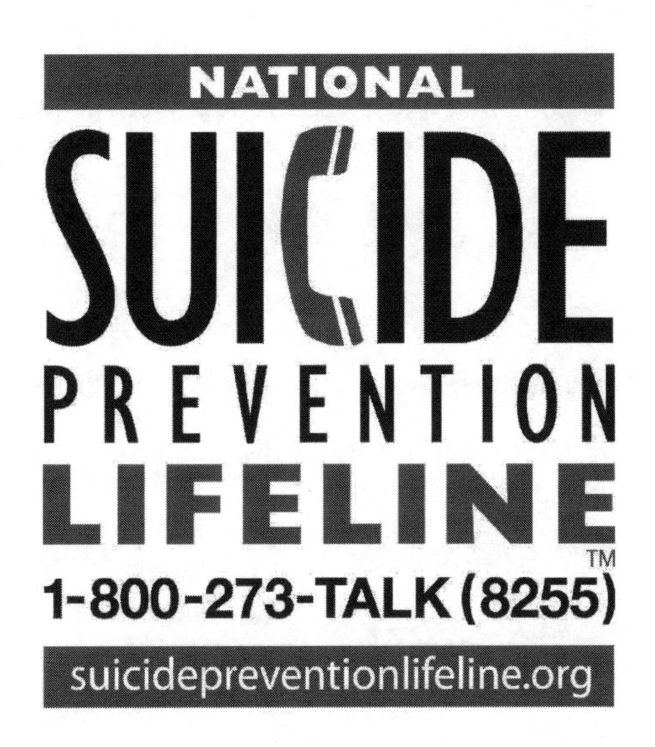

Alcohol Abuse and Drug Addictions

Alcohol Abuse

Alcohol remains the most widely abused substance among America's youth, with a higher percentage of youth ages 12 to 20 using more alcohol in the past month (25.1%) than tobacco (19.6%) or illicit drugs (14.9%).

The extent of alcohol consumption by those younger than the legal drinking age of 21 is a serious threat to both public health and public safety. Underage drinking and associated problems have profound negative consequences for underage drinkers, their families, their communities, and society.

Underage drinking contributes to a wide range of costly health and social problems, including:

- ✓ Motor vehicle crashes (greatest single mortality risk for underage drinkers)
- ✓ Suicide
- ✓ Interpersonal violence (for example, homicides, assaults, rapes)
- ✓ Unintentional injuries, such as burns, falls, and drowning
- ✓ Brain impairment
- ✓ Alcohol dependence
- ✓ Risky sexual activity
- ✓ Academic problems
- ✓ Alcohol and drug poisoning

On average, alcohol is a factor in the deaths of approximately 4,700 youths in the United States per year, shortening their lives by an average of 60 years.
Research shows that parents are the leading influence on their child's decisions about alcohol. Many parents make efforts to ensure that their children understand that underage drinking is illegal and can carry negative health and academic

consequences. Alcohol use among college students, including among those who are under age 21, is common and can have serious negative consequences.

Activity #4: Alcohol Intake Assessment

Let's Reflect! Without sharing or writing your response down, think about how much alcohol you consume on a daily or weekly basis.

- ✓ Would you classify yourself as a non- drinker, light drinker, moderate drinker, or heavy drinker?
- ✓ Do you think your drinking behavior is risky?
- ✓ If you chose to drink, think of ways you can ensure you are doing so in the safest way possible.
    - i.e. never getting behind the wheel after drinking (or getting in a car with someone else who has been drinking) etc.

Drug Addictions

Many people don't understand why or how themselves or other people become addicted to drugs. They may mistakenly think that those who use drugs lack moral principles or willpower and that they could stop their drug use simply by choosing to. In reality, drug addiction is a complex disease, and quitting usually takes more than good intentions or a strong will. Drugs change the brain in ways that make quitting hard, even for those who want to. Fortunately, researchers know more than ever about how drugs affect the brain and have found treatments that can help people recover from drug addiction and lead productive lives.

What Is Drug Addiction?

Addiction is a chronic disease characterized by drug seeking and use that is compulsive, or difficult to control, despite harmful consequences. The initial decision to take drugs is voluntary for most people, but repeated drug use can lead to brain changes that challenge an addicted person's self-control and interfere with their ability to resist intense urges to take drugs. These brain changes can be persistent, which is why drug addiction is considered a "relapsing" disease—people in recovery from drug use disorders are at increased risk for returning to drug use even after years of not taking the drug.

It's common for a person to relapse, but relapse doesn't mean that treatment doesn't work. As with other chronic health conditions, treatment should be ongoing and should be adjusted based on how someone responds. Treatment plans need to be reviewed often and modified to fit the patient's changing needs.

Can Drug Addiction Be Cured or Prevented?

As with most other chronic diseases, such as diabetes, asthma, or heart disease, treatment for drug addiction generally does not have a cure. However, addiction is treatable and can be successfully managed. People who are recovering from an addiction will be at risk for relapse for years and possibly for their whole lives. Research shows that combining addiction treatment medicines with behavioral therapy ensures the best chance of success for most patients. Treatment approaches tailored to each patient's drug use patterns and any co-occurring medical, mental, and social problems can lead to continued recovery.

Types of Drug Addictions

Marijuana

Marijuana (cannabis) is the most commonly used illicit substance. This drug impairs short-term memory and learning, the ability to focus, and coordination. It also increases heart rate, can harm the lungs, and may increase the risk of psychosis in vulnerable people. Research suggests that when regular marijuana use begins in the teen years, addiction is more likely: 1 in 6 users, compared to 1 in 9 among adults. In addition, recent research suggests that heavy cannabis use that starts in the teen years is associated with declines in IQ scores in adulthood.

Prescription and Over-the-Counter Medications

Prescription medications and some over-the-counter medications are increasingly being abused (used in ways other than intended or without a prescription). This practice can lead to addiction, and in some cases, overdose. Among the most disturbing aspects of this emerging trend is its prevalence among teenagers and young adults, as well as the common misperception that because these are used medically or prescribed by physicians, they are safe even when not used as intended. Commonly abused classes of prescription drugs include opioid painkillers, stimulants, and depressants.

OPIOIDS are usually prescribed for pain relief. Commonly prescribed opioids include hydrocodone (i.e., Vicodin®), oxycodone (i.e., OxyContin®), morphine, fentanyl, and codeine. In the United States, more people now die from opioid painkiller overdoses than from heroin and cocaine combined.

STIMULANTS include methylphenidate (Ritalin®, Concerta®, Focalin®, and Metadate®) and amphetamines (Adderall®, Dexedrine®) are stimulants commonly prescribed for attention-deficit hyperactivity disorder (ADHD).

DEPRESSANTS are usually prescribed to promote sleep or to reduce anxiety. As measured by national surveys, depressants are often categorized as sedatives or tranquilizers. Sedatives primarily include barbiturates (i.e., phenobarbitol) but also include sleep medications such as Ambien® and Lunesta®. Tranquilizers primarily include benzodiazepines such as Valium® and Xanax®, but also include muscle relaxants and other anti-anxiety medications.

Another common mixture that is made by using prescription medications is known as "Syrup," "purple drank," "sizzurp," or "lean". These mixtures describe soda combined with prescription-strength cough syrup containing codeine and promethazine, which are available by prescription only. Users may also flavor the mixture with hard candies. Drinking this combination has become increasingly popular among some celebrities and youth in several areas of the country. Codeine is an opioid that can produce relaxation and euphoria when consumed in sufficient quantities. Promethazine is an antihistamine that also acts as a sedative.

Commonly abused over-the-counter drugs include cold medicines containing dextromethorphan (DMX), a cough suppressant. Products containing DMX can be sold as cough syrups, gel capsules, and pills. They are frequently abused and is referred to as "robo-tripping" or "skittling."

Heroin

Heroin is a substance that is both illegal and extremely addictive. The substance derives from opium from the poppy plant before it is refined to morphine, then further chemically modified to become heroin. Despite its deserved negative reputation for its high risks, heroin continues to be a commonly abused drug in the U.S.

Signs and Symptoms of Heroin Use

Signs and symptoms of heroin abuse will depend on how much, how often, and how long it has been abused.

IMMEDIATE SYMPTOMS	DELAYED SYMPTOMS	SIGNS OF LONG-TERM USE
Some users report immediate negative symptoms from drug: • Nausea • Vomiting • Itching • Dry mouth	Following the immediate effects of heroin, another set of symptoms begin to occur that involve the body slowing down and being less active and alert. These signs of heroin use include. • Feeling drowsy and sleepy for hours • Having a foggy mental state • Slowed breathing • Slowed heart rate • "Nodding" where user will alternate between periods of being awake and asleep.	With continued use over a period of time, person abusing heroin may exhibit other signs like: • Needle marks and bruising on injection sites • Skin problems like abscesses and infections. • Heart Problems • Disease in organs including the liver and kidneys. • Collapsed veins from repeated injections.

Opioid Overdoses in Connecticut

Similar to other states, Connecticut has had a rise in drug overdoses as the opioid addiction epidemic continues to increase. Fatal overdoses increased in 2016 to 917 fatal overdoses from 729 in 2015. Figures for fatal overdoses are from the result of opioid overdoes and do not include alcohol overdoses.

The following towns had the most residents die of opioid overdoses in 2016:

- ✓ Hartford: 62
- ✓ Bridgeport: 49
- ✓ New Haven: 44
- ✓ Bristol: 35
- ✓ New Britain: 35
- ✓ Waterbury 33
- ✓ Norwich: 24
- ✓ Meriden: 24
- ✓ West Haven: 21
- ✓ Stratford: 20

Recently, legislation has passed laws in an attempt to reduce the opioid epidemic. For example, a prescription monitoring program was implemented to restrict "doctor shopping" for multiple opioid prescriptions. There are now armed police or other first emergency responders with naloxone to reverse overdoses in the field. Naloxone can now be prescribed by pharmacists.

A law passed last year to limit initial prescription for opioids to 7 days. After that, it's up to a physician if the patient needs more. Exceptions are in place for chronic pain, cancer-associated pain, and palliative care.

Chapter Summary

- ✓ Many factors contribute to disruptions in your mental well-being, including: biological factors, such as genes or brain chemistry; life experiences, such as trauma or abuse; family history of mental health problems
- ✓ Depression does not have a single cause. It can be triggered by a life crisis, physical illness or something else—but it can also occur spontaneously. Scientists conclude several factors can contribute, such as: trauma, genetics, life circumstances, brain changes, medical conditions, and drug/alcohol abuse.
- ✓ A few complimentary ways to help improve anxiety and depression include: Stress and relaxation techniques, Meditation, Yoga, and Acupuncture.
- ✓ Eating disorders are more than just one type. They are a group of related conditions that involve extreme food and body weight issues; however, each has unique symptoms that separate it from the others.
- ✓ PTSD affects 3.5% of the U.S. adult population—about 7.7 million Americans—but women are more likely to develop the condition than men. About 37% of those cases are classified as severe.
- ✓ Suicide rates among college students have increased by 200 percent since the 1950s, and today, suicide is one of the leading causes of death among college and university students in the United States.

- ✓ Attempts at suicide and death by suicide are most common in college students who: are depressed; are either under the influence of substances or have a substance use problem; have made a previous attempt; have a family history of a mood disorder such as depression or bipolar disorder; and are struggling with a history of trauma.
- ✓ Underage drinking and associated problems have profound negative consequences for underage drinkers, their families, their communities, and society
- ✓ Drug addiction is a complex disease. Drugs change the brain in ways that make quitting hard, even for those who want to. If you struggle with a drug addition, seek help as soon as possible.

Chapter Review Questions

1) What are the differences between mental disorders and mental illnesses?
2) Identify the warning signs of significant mental health disturbances.
3) Detail the most recent statistics on mental illness.
4) Know the most recent statistics on depression and anxiety disorders.
5) Detail the recommended treatment methods for depression, anxiety disorders, and PTSD.
6) Identify the warning signs of teenage suicide.
7) Describe the warning signs and treatment methods for people with eating disorders.
8) Outline what you learned about alcohol abuse and drug addictions from the book chapter.

References

National Alliance on Mental Illness: **www.nami.org**

Students Against Depression: **http://studentsagainstdepression.org/**

National Eating Disorders Association **www.nationaleatingdisorders.org/**

Suicide Statistics: Suicide Prevention Resource Center

Alcohol Abuse Statistics: **www.samhsa.gov/school-campus-health/substance-use-mental-health**

Drug Additions: **www.drugabuse.gov/publications/drugfacts/understanding-drug-use-addiction**

Marijuana: **www.drugabuse.gov/drugs-abuse/marijuana.**

Heroin Abuse: **www.drugabuse.com/library/heroin-abuse/**

Connecticut Heroin Epidemic: **patch.com/connecticut/newcanaan/ct-heroin-epidemic-interactive-map-deaths-town-0**

Prescription drug abuse and related health consequences: **www.drugabuse.gov/drugs-abuse/prescription-drugs-cold-medicines**

Chapter 5

Positive Lifestyle and Wellness

By Jim Malley, PhD

Chapter Objectives

After reading this chapter, students should be able to:

- ✓ Understand the concepts of 'flourishing' and 'happiness' and to distinguish the differences between the two;
- ✓ Identify the difference between an intrinsic value and an extrinsic value;
- ✓ Understand the concepts of contemplation, meditation and mindfulness;
- ✓ Recognize the important tasks the brain is responsible for and the importance of keeping our brains healthy;
- ✓ Recognize how early childhood life impacts individuals across their lifespan and learn how an individual who has experienced a traumatic childhood can improve their mental health; and
- ✓ Understand the importance of compassion and know the difference between compassion and empathy.

Positive Lifestyle and Wellness

"Educating the mind without educating the heart is no education at all." - Aristotle

Flourishing and Happiness

Activity #1: Happiness Reflection

Before beginning this chapter, take a few moments to reflect and then write down 3 things that would make you the most happy and fulfilled in life. When you are finished, write your 3 things on the whiteboard. After everyone has written their statements on the whiteboard, carry on a class discussion facilitated by your professor.

- ✓ What statements did you agree with?
- ✓ What statements surprised you?
- ✓ What items might be missing?
- ✓ What common themes did you see?

This chapter explores several aspects of positive mental health and wellbeing that provide the seeds to human happiness and flourishing. The material may seem a bit new and different to you. You might even think it is a bit "hippy-dippy" because it comes from ancient contemplative practices and emerging new research about the plastic nature of the human brain.

We will explore how the practices of (1) contemplation, (2) mindfulness, and (3) meditation are becoming mainstream in contemporary culture and how they can help us become more caring, compassionate and healthier human beings. Lastly, we will explore one of society's greatest unaddressed public health problems - the mistreatment of children, and how mindfulness can play an important role in lessening the effects of early childhood stress and trauma.

The definition of flourish is "to grow or develop in a healthy or vigorous way, especially as the result of a particularly favorable environment" (google.dic). We know, for example, that when flowers grow into their full radiant beauty, it is because they were nurtured in just the right kind of environment. This chapter attempts to explore the question: what kind of environment does it take to help humans become fully human? It's a critical question when we consider the full range of possible behaviors that humans have exacted upon the world throughout history: from peacemaking to terrorism, from the creation of extraordinary works of art to the trashing of the natural world. Thus, understanding the connection between healthy human development and one's environment is critically important.

It was this nexus that was of supreme interest to Abraham Maslow (1971), one of the world's best-known psychologists and creator of the concept of self-actualization. He viewed the relationship between the person and the society as the problem of big problems: "*the first and overarching Big Problem is to make the Good Person. We must have better human beings or else it is quite possible that we may all be wiped out…" (p. 19).* But, to make the good person, he insisted, we must have a good society.

Part of Maslow's concern rested with his recognition that while society was rapidly progressing technologically, it remained light years behind in social development. Writing some time prior to his death in 1970, he worried that society was headed in the wrong direction as it approached the 21st century. He wrote:

> *Another way of expressing my uneasiness is to point out that much of this talk about the year 2000 is at a merely material level, for example, of industrialization, modernization, increasing affluence, greater possession of more things. (*p. 24).

Maslow (1971) believed that rather than emphasizing having, consuming, and achieving, a *Good Society* was one that fostered human flourishing. Such a society would need to be based on a foundation of transcendent values such as love, truth, goodness, beauty, and justice.

Carl Rogers (1959), another famous psychologist who shared much of Maslow's thinking, suggested that mental anxieties and a loss of self-worth occurred when there was a gap between what one believes and how one behaves in the world. He referred to this as the need for congruence, i.e. to behave in according with one's values and ideals.

That need for congruence applies not just to individuals but also to whole societies. This sentiment was beautifully articulated by Robert F. Kennedy, Attorney General of the United States, in his famous speech on the importance of values at the University of Kansas (Kennedy, 1968). Speaking of the country's preoccupation with the gross national product, he said:

"The gross national product does not allow for the health of our children, the quality of their education, or the joy of their play. It does not include the beauty of our poetry or the strength of our marriages; the intelligence of our public debate or the integrity of our public officials. It measures neither wit nor courage; neither our wisdom nor our teaching; neither our compassion nor our devotion to our country; it measures everything, in short, except that which makes life worthwhile."

Sadly, Kennedy was assassinated only 3 months later, on June 5, 1968, robbing him of the opportunity to promulgate his views on the importance of values.

The Nobel-Laureate economist, Gunnar Myrdal, expressed one of the most disturbing examples of our nation's failure to live according to its espoused values. In his book, *An American Dilemma*, Myrdal pointed to the cruel oppression and mistreatment of black people by a nation that believed all people were created equal. Almost 75 years later, it is a problem that continues to tear at the soul of America.

Rokeach (cited in Crompton, 2010) defined human values as psychological representations of what we believe to be important in life. Because we believe values are important, they hold emotional appeal and we try to attain them. Crompton made a distinction between intrinsic or self-transcendent values, and extrinsic or self-enhancing values. The two sets of values are almost diametrically opposed. For example, striving for personal wealth or fame would be extrinsic values since they are self-enhancing. Crompton cited studies showing a strong interest in financial success was associated with lower empathy, more manipulative tendencies, and a higher tolerance for social inequality.

Contrariwise, intrinsic values stem from a sense of community and a desire to make the world a better place through civic action. Which values a person endorses may be due to a range of factors including upbringing, social norms or the media. For example, the media and advertising industries tend to promote materialistic values at the expense of socially beneficial values.

Positive Psychology

What values make life worthwhile and foster human happiness and flourishing? That was a question that was asked by psychologist, Martin Seligman (cited in Lopez et al, 2015), who is credited with developing the field of positive psychology. The field of positive psychology was created as a reaction to psychology's long held preoccupation with psychological illness instead of psychological health.

Positive psychology is defined as "the science and applications related to the study of psychological strengths and positive emotions" (p. 18). Peterson and Seligman (2004) identified the following 6 overarching strengths or virtues that undergird the very best of humanity: wisdom, knowledge, courage, humanity, justice, temperance, and transcendence. It is not a coincidence that these strengths also correlate with measures of happiness and life satisfaction (Lopez et al., 2015).

Happiness

The quality of human happiness has been explored since ancient Greece. Aristotle used the word *eudemonia*, which could be translated as either happiness or human flourishing. In his *Nicomachean Ethics*, Aristotle said that eudaimonia was the highest good for human beings and that it consisted of living well and realizing one's fullest potential (Apostle & Gerson, 1991).

The world's longest running study on happiness is still being carried out by the Harvard Medical School. The Harvard Study of Adult Development (Powell, 2017), began in 1938 when the researchers began tracking 268 sophomores. One of the recruits included John F. Kennedy who would eventually go on to become President of the United States. The study continues to this day and was expanded to include 1300 of the men's offspring.

Of the study's 4 major findings:

- ✓ A happy childhood has long-lasting effects including better physical health well into old age.
- ✓ People with difficult childhoods can make up for them in midlife.
- ✓ Learning how to cope well with stress has a lifelong payoff.
- ✓ It's the quality of your relationships that really matter.

Activity #2: What Makes a Good Life?

View and discuss the TED talk online under the title:

- ✓ "*What makes a good life?*" by Robert Waldinger.

What is most important to living a worthwhile life?

Come to class prepared to discuss the key ingredients to living a good life.

While education is almost exclusively focused on learning about the outer world, there is growing evidence that exploring our inner worlds may be the truer path to discovering happiness and human flourishing. Self-exploration through contemplative practices has been shown to promote increased self-awareness and the ability to manage our thoughts and emotions and enjoy healthy relationships. The following section explores contemplative practices including mindfulness and meditation.

Contemplation

"The unexamined life is not worth living." - Socrates

Contemplative practices ask life's big questions: *What is life all about? Why are we here? What is our purpose?*

The word contemplation is an overarching term that refers to a variety of ways in which people explore their inner lives through reflection, introspection, and meditation. While most Western education tends to emphasize learning about the external world, contemplation takes us inside to explore our interior worlds as we seek to live fuller, richer, and happier lives. Of course, we need to take courses like math, science, history, and geography to learn about the outside world and build a knowledge base to prepare for a meaningful career. These kinds of courses provide us with valuable information that helps us to know about the world, but they don't necessarily prepare us to learn how to "**be**" in the world. We need to go inside to do that. Carl Jung, the renowned psychoanalyst said it this way: *"Your vision will become clear only when you can look into your own heart. Who looks outside, dreams; who looks inside, awakes."* (Brainy Quote.com)

The Center for Contemplative Mind in Society (Barbezat & Bush, 2014) suggests that contemplation represents an effort to find out what is most meaningful in life. This often requires deep concentration, self-reflection, and finding clarity by quieting the mind to achieve a state of calmness amid a noisy and busy world. Henry David

Thoreau was perhaps one of the most well-known contemplatives. He was part of the so-called transcendental movement in the mid 1800's that was based on a belief that society and its various institutions were corrupting the true meaning of life. Transcendentalists believed in the importance of one's inner spiritual life. The movement was probably best captured by Thoreau's (1995) famous lines from Walden:

> *I went to the woods because I wished to live deliberately, to front only the essential facts of life, and see if I could not learn what it had to teach, and not, when I came to die, discover that I had not lived.*

Many contemplative practices depicted in the image on the next page (Figure 1) have their roots in a variety of centuries-old religious practices including prayer and pilgrimages. Contemplation was also at the heart of inquiry by the great philosophers and wisdom seekers like Plato, Aristotle, and Socrates in ancient Greece. Unlike contemporary education that focuses primarily on cognitive pursuits, education at that time was more concerned with the whole person - mind, body and soul. Reflecting on current trends Barbezat and Bush (2014) remarked: *"Somehow we have lost our way in higher education and abandoned our mission to create lives of purpose and strong ethical and creative minds"* (p. xv).

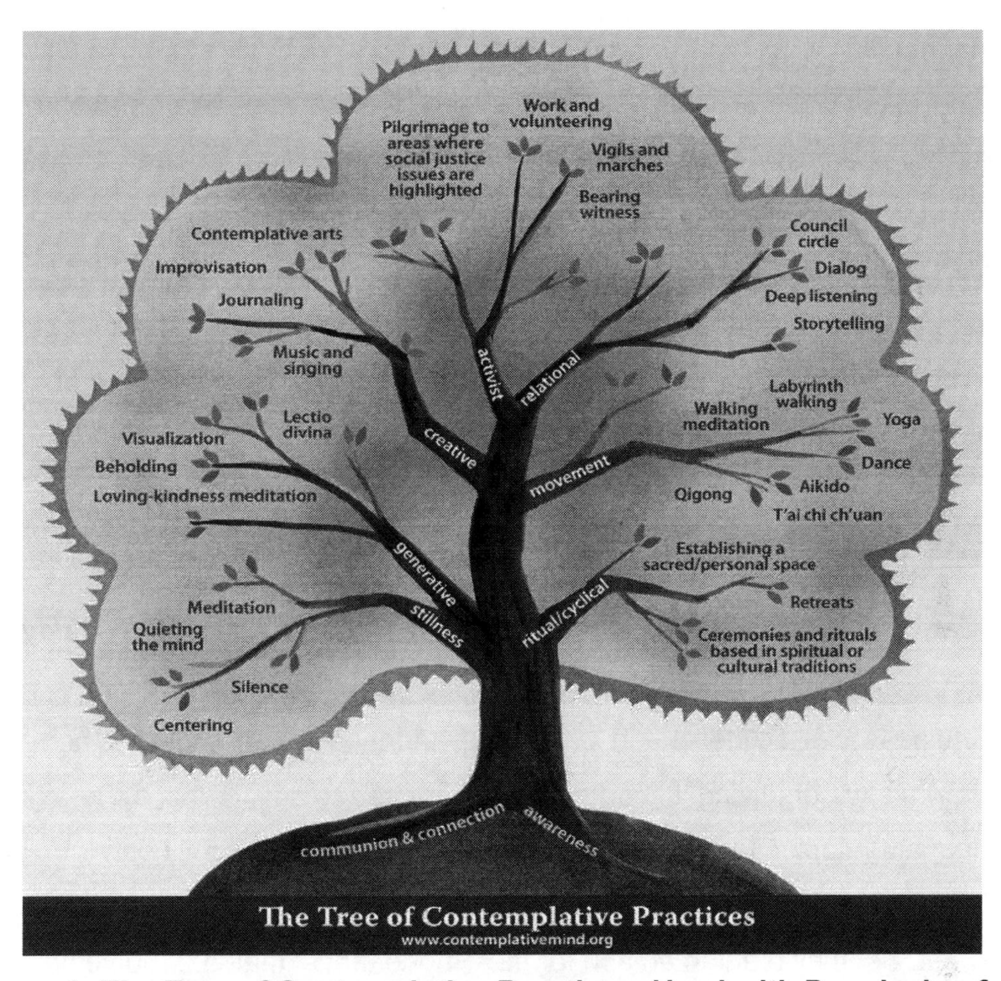

Figure 1: The Tree of Contemplative Practices. Used with Permission from Center for the Contemplative Mind in Society

The author, Parker Palmer (cited in Barbezat et al., 2014), suggested that the increased interest in contemplative practices is a reaction to the objectivist model of education that has dominated teaching and learning. Referring to Socrates' famous dictum to know oneself, he pointed out that people who do not know themselves are much more prone to damaging themselves or others. Palmer noted that contemplative practices have become increasingly important at a time when education must support the causes of truth, love, and justice: *"students whose minds and hearts have been formed by contemplation of self, as well as world are much more likely to become the kind of ethical actors we need at a time when basic human values are so widely threatened"* (p. ix).

Contemplation is also regarded by many to be the only sure pathway to wisdom. A person might have a great deal of knowledge about the external world, even be a *Jeopardy* champion, but still lack wisdom. Contemplation requires the willingness to go inward even if at first it seems scary. The downside of not "knowing ourselves" is that we become easy prey to other people's thinking, what Palmer (2014) called, "the myriad pitchmen of meaning who con us into buying their cut-rate, bogus remedies for emptiness and fear" (p. 62). The advertising industry is much more successful with people who are unable to think for themselves.

Mindfulness

Do human beings ever realize life while they are living it? – Emily Webb

Mindfulness can be described as paying attention to life on a moment-to-moment basis while we are living it. You might be tempted to say, "What's the big deal about paying attention?" Two Harvard psychologists, Matthew Killingsworth and Daniel Gilbert (Powell, 2010), were curious about how much we really pay attention in each moment. So, they created an app for the iPhone that signaled 2250 volunteers to stop at various times when prompted during the day and answer the following questions: 1) What were they doing? 2) What were they thinking about? 3) Were they happy at the time?

Analyzing up to 250,000 data points, the researchers found that 46.9% of the time, subjects were thinking about something else other than what they were doing. In other words, for almost half of their awake time, the subjects' minds were wandering. Perhaps they were thinking about something in the past or the future, but they were not engaged in the present moment. Furthermore, researchers found subjects were less happy when their attention was pulled away from what they were doing, leading them to conclude: a wandering mind is an unhappy mind.

Isn't it shocking to realize that, if we were fortunate to live to 100 years old, for almost 50 years we wouldn't have been paying attention to what we were doing?

Based on the findings of this study, one could argue that all humans have a bit of an attention deficit disorder.

Activity #3: Your Wandering Mind

Do you have a wandering mind? To find out, try this exercise.

1) Sit in an upright position, back straight, with feet planted firmly on the floor.
2) Close your eyes or, if you prefer, soften and lower your gaze.
3) Take an in breath (about 5 sec), hold for 3 sec, breathe out (about 5 sec)
4) After each in and out breath - silently count to yourself "one."
5) Continue with your second breath and count "two" - and so on for 10 breaths
6) As you breathe, notice if you are visited by any uninvited thoughts.
7) After your 10th breath, record your findings. Did you have any thoughts? How many?
8) What is your conclusion? Did your mind tend to wander?

Once an ancient contemplative practice associated with many different religions, mindfulness has become mainstream in contemporary American culture. It has found its way into corporate life, professional sports, and in health and education. The on-line *Merriam-Webster Dictionary* defines mindfulness as: *the practice of maintaining a nonjudgmental state of heightened or complete awareness of one's thoughts, emotions, or experiences on a moment-to-moment basis.*

Jon Kabat-Zinn (2005) is often credited with secularizing mindfulness in Western culture, something that was previously considered to be a Buddhist practice. A student of Buddhism and yoga, Kabat-Zinn was a Professor of Medicine at the UMASS Medical Center in Worcester, Massachusetts. It occurred to him that mindfulness might be of benefit to patients that experienced chronic medical conditions, stress, and pain. This led him to create an 8-week Mindfulness Based Stress Reduction (MBSR) program that led to significant improvements in his patients. Since it began in 1979 MBSR is now practiced in hospitals and clinics all over the world.

Mindfulness in K-12 Education

Mindfulness is also being increasingly used in K-12 school systems to help both teachers and children reduce stress-levels, become more emotionally self-regulated, and sharpen their attentional focus (Black & Fernando, 2013). Mindfulness is an important tool in social and emotional training programs that are growing rapidly in K-12 public schools throughout the country.

CCSU's own School of Education and Professional Studies (SEPS) has established a Center for Social and Emotional Learning (SEL) that consults with local school systems in the use of SEL programs, including those that are mindfulness based. A number of schools in Connecticut are experimenting with mindfulness in the classroom. As one example, the Breakthrough Magnet School in Hartford has had a fully implemented mindfulness program for more than 3 years. In 2015 the Breakthrough Magnet School was voted as the "best magnet school in the country" (Medina, 2015).

Meditation

While mindfulness might be thought of as a way to be more present in our own lives, meditation can be thought of as a way to get better at being mindful, just like lifting weights is a way to get stronger. In this section we will discuss research that has shown that a regular practice of meditation can strengthen the brain's neural circuitry that improves one's ability to pay attention on a moment by moment basis.

There is growing evidence that meditation is becoming more mainstream in society. Consider the following:

- *Time Magazine* (Feb. 2014) featured a cover story on *The Mindful Revolution*
- *Scientific American* (Nov. 2014) featured a cover story about the "*Neuroscience of Meditation*"

- An article in the *Wall Street Journal* (Feb. 2015) asked, *Can Mindfulness help students do better in school?*
- In December 2014, the newscaster, Anderson Cooper, disclosed on 60 Minutes that he was a regular meditator.
- Tim Ryan, U.S. Congressman from Ohio published his book *A Mindful Nation: How a Simple Practice Can Help Us Reduce Stress, Improve Performance and Recapture the American Spirit* (2012)

SAMPLING OF PEOPLE WHO MEDITATE: Kobe Bryant, Bill Ford, LeBron James, Ellen DeGeneres, Katy Perry, Jerry Seinfeld, Michael Jordan, Barry Zito, Ricky Williams, Anderson Cooper, Phil Jackson, Jennifer Anston, Amy Schumer, Misty May-Treanor, Oprah, Dan Harris, Congressman Tim Ryan, Mark Bertolini.
SAMPLING OF CORPORATIONS THAT ENCOURAGE MEDITATION: Aetna, eBay, Target, Apple, Yahoo, Google, Boeing, Facebook, Twitter, Green Mountain Coffee, NASA, Texas Instruments, Ford Motor, General Mills, Department of Defense, Kaiser Permanente, Hughes Aircraft.

Activity #4: Athletes and Meditation

Meditation is practiced by many world-class athletes. View the following YouTube videos:

- ✓ *George Mumford on How to Be Mindful*
- ✓ *Kobe Bryant and Phil Jackson on Meditation*

Be prepared to discuss in class.

How Do We Meditate?

The process of meditation is quite simple. Because meditation is a personal choice it is always done by invitation. Should any students prefer not to meditate they can be invited to just sit quietly. The instruction is to sit in a comfortable position with your feet firmly planted on the floor and your back straight. You can sit cross-legged on a cushion, the posture that is most commonly depicted in pictures of people meditating. But this requires a bit of flexibility; for those less flexible it is perfectly okay to just sit in a chair. When I first started having students meditate at the beginning of each class, some of the more fatigued students would instinctively lay their heads on the desk. I would have to remind them that that was more of a sleeping position than a meditating position.

Once seated, you then close your eyes or, if you prefer, soften and lower your gaze just in front of your feet. Then bring your attention to your breath, noticing each in-breath and each out-breath. Notice how, with each breath, your chest or belly rises and falls. As you pay attention to your breath, you will inevitably be visited by a thought, even if the thought was uninvited. Recall, that above we learned that our minds tend to wander and that it is just part of being human. When you notice that you have wandered to a thought or an idea, simply notice that with curiosity and without judgment and return to your breath. Rosenberg (1998) has described the meditation process in the following way:

> *The whole process is meditation: being with the breathing, drifting away, seeing that we've drifted away, gently coming back. It is extremely important to come back without blame, without judgment, without a feeling of failure. If you have to come back a thousand times in a five -minute period of sitting, just do it. It's not a problem unless you make it into one (p.34).*

Sitting and focusing on one's breath seems quite simple, doesn't it? But, maintaining a regular, disciplined practice is anything but, especially in our fast-paced world, when just sitting and breathing seems like such an anomaly.

One helpful suggestion to reinforce a regular practice is to occasionally join with others in group meditations and/or attend meditation retreats. You are also welcome to join the weekly **Moment-to-Moment meditations** that take place right on the CCSU campus through RECentral.

Activity #5: Guided Meditation

Participate as a class in the following 14-minute Guided Meditation by meditation teacher Tara Brach on YouTube:

- ✓ *Tara Brach Leads a Guided Meditation: Opening and Calming*

Simply follow the instructions and be aware there will be periods of silence in which you just sit quietly focusing on your breath. If you prefer to opt out, simply sit quietly and you can view the changing scenes on the You Tube video. You are also free to stop anytime during the meditation. The end of the meditation will be signaled by the ringing of 3 bells.

Hold a class discussion. How did you experience the meditation?

What are the Benefits of Meditation?

You might be asking - *what are the benefits that might ensue if I meditate on a regular basis?* Emma Seppala (2017), Science Director for the Stanford Medical School Center for Compassion and Altruism Research and Education (CCARE) cited research on the multiple health benefits of mindfulness practice including reductions in stress, anxiety, and depression, improved immune system functioning, and less emotional reactivity. Here are some of the benefits she found scientific research for:

It Boosts Your HAPPINESS

- ✓ Increases Positive Emotion
- ✓ Decreases Depression
- ✓ Decreases Anxiety
- ✓ Decreases Stress

It Boosts Your SOCIAL LIFE

- ✓ Increases social connection & emotional intelligence
- ✓ Makes you more compassionate
- ✓ Makes you feel less lonely

It Boosts Your Self-Control

- ✓ Improves your ability to regulate your emotions
- ✓ Improves your ability to introspect

Two prominent behavioral scientists Daniel Goleman, a psychologist, and Richard Davidson, a neuroscientist, co-authored the recently published book, *Altered Traits: Science Reveals How Meditation Changes Your Mind, Brain, and Body (2017).* After combing through the myriad of studies on mindfulness they concluded, that when practiced consistently over time, meditation can engender the following benefits:

- ✓ Meditation can improve our resiliency to stress
- ✓ Meditation can increase our capacity for compassion toward others by decreasing our focus on ourselves.
- ✓ Remarkably, meditation might even improve our health and increase our longevity.

Once rooted in many religious disciplines that go back more than two thousand years, contemplation, mindfulness, and meditation have become mainstream in the health and education professions due to their demonstrated benefits in promoting human health and well-being. In particular, neuroscience research has shown that mindfulness practices can promote human resiliency, protect people from the deleterious effects of toxic stress, increase one's capacity for happiness and compassion, and increase one's lifespan.

Can Meditation Increase Compassion?

Activity #6: Test of Compassion

Imagine that you walk into the waiting room of a doctor's office. There are only 3 chairs in the room and two of them are occupied. You sit in the one available chair. Then a woman enters the room using crutches and appearing to be in pain. The people in the other 2 chairs seem oblivious to the woman.

What would you do? Discuss your response.

The above scenario was from a study conducted by researchers from Harvard and Northeastern University (Condon et al., 2013). Researchers were interested in examining whether meditation increased compassionate behavior. The 2 people in the chairs and the woman with crutches were actually associates to the study. Researchers invited two groups of subjects to participate; one group completed an 8-week training program in meditation. The other served as the control group.

The results found that only 15 percent of the non-meditators offered to help the suffering woman compared to 50 percent of the meditators. The almost 5-fold difference between meditators and non-meditators suggests that meditation significantly increases compassionate behavior. Other studies with people who participated in a particular type of meditation training called "loving-kindness meditation" actually showed structural changes the meditators' brains. The meditators also donated higher amounts to charities compared to non-meditators (Galante, 2016; Weng et al., 2013).

These studies seem to scientifically validate the Dalai Lama's (2011) contention that compassion is the foundation for human well-being and that we could change the world by paying more attention to what he referred to as education of the heart:

> *I am hopeful that a time will come when we can take it for granted that children will learn as a part of their school curriculum, the indispensability of inner values such as love, compassion, justice, and forgiveness (p. 187).*

Compassion may be one of the most important qualities for insuring human survival and well-being. Although compassion resides as a potential in everyone, it must be cultivated just as a flower needs to be nurtured from a seed. Studies suggest that a regular meditation is one way to increase the human capacity for compassion.

CCSU: A Campus of Compassion

Did you know that CCSU has been designated by the International Charter for Compassion as a "university of compassion?" The impetus for the compassion campaign came in 2012 when faculty learned that the Charter for Compassion had designated our sister school, Western Connecticut State University, as a "university of compassion" following a visit from His Holiness the Dalai Lama to its campus.

Following a three-year campaign, the CCSU Faculty Senate voted unanimously in 2015 to endorse the Campus of Compassion campaign and recommended the appointment of a Presidential Committee on Compassion. Following are some of the reasons that the Faculty Senate cited in their resolution:

1) As leaders in an academic community, it is our responsibility to role model behavior that fosters mutual respect and provides a safe environment for all human beings regardless of race, gender, religion, age, sexual orientation, disability, and socioeconomic status

2) Scientific research has shown that compassion helps to build human connection and a sense of community and plays a critical role in childhood development and the emotional health and well-being of all humans.
3) Service is a strong part of CCSU's heritage in which students, faculty, staff, and alumni engage with others to improve their community.

Furthermore, the Faculty Senate concluded that as a regional comprehensive university, CCSU had the responsibility to find solutions to the enormous problems facing the world including terrorism, violence, extreme poverty, and environmental deterioration. It was acknowledged that even in our own state, with strong and vibrant communities, Connecticut is also home to pockets of extreme poverty, epidemic levels of drug and alcohol addiction, sex trafficking, and one of the most horrific school shootings in the world. CCSU is committed to finding solutions to these serious problems that contribute to human suffering.

Compassion versus Empathy

There is often confusion about the qualitative difference between empathy and compassion. While they are both desirable human qualities, there is an important distinction. Empathy is the ability of a person to emotionally sense what another person is feeling at a given time. To empathize is to almost experience the same feeling of the other, be it sadness, happiness, or joy. Compassion, however, is a specific response to someone else's suffering. You not only have empathy for that person, but there is an action component - you want to see the person relieved of the suffering (Dalai Lama, 2011).

Armstrong (2010) argued that compassion might be the one quality that best defines what it means to be a mature human being: "instead of being motivated by self-interest, a truly humane person [is] consistently oriented toward others" (p. 10). To be compassionate, is to be more human.

His Holiness the Dalai Lama (2011) believes that many of the world's problems such as alcoholism, drug abuse, domestic abuse, and family breakdown stem from our failure to cultivate compassion. Perhaps "cultivate" is the operative word here. While the capacity for compassion may reside in every human being, it doesn't just emerge naturally; it has to be exercised just like a muscle has to be exercised to be strong. As mentioned above, a regular meditation practice has been shown to be one way to increase compassion.

Is Compassion Manly?

Most people would likely agree that compassion is a desirable trait in men. After all, most men are law abiding, good husbands, good fathers, and good citizens. And, some men like Gandhi, Martin Luther King, Nelson Mandela, the Dalai Lama, and Bishop Tutu have been living examples of compassion. However, there is a strong countervailing attitude in American culture that qualities like kindness and compassion are signs of weakness, in other words, not masculine. This stereotypical image of hyper-masculine behavior glorifies physical strength, aggression and sexuality (Mosher et al., 1988) that is perpetuated by the media.

This was a concern expressed by Joe Ehrmann, an NFL player, whose life story is chronicled in *Seasons of Life* by Jeffrey Marx (2004). Ehrmann was a defensive lineman who captained the Baltimore Colts and made the Pro Bowl in 1978. After he retired, his passion as an ordained minister has been to destroy what he described as the three lies of false masculinity, i.e., that manhood is best measured by athletic ability, sexual conquest, and economic success. Ehrmann said that these myths contribute to a life of failure for so many men, and exact a terrible price on society measured in terms of destroyed relationships, violence, and drug addiction

Ehrmann's concern is shared by others. Robert Sapolsky (2017), professor of biology and neurology at Stanford University, and author of *Behave: The Biology of Humans at Our Best and Worst* observed that male violence is pervasive in the world. A casual acquaintance with the news seems to support the contention that most atrocities, i.e., gun violence including mass shootings, terrorism, rapes and sexual violence, domestic violence, drug cartel related murders, and youth gangs are predominantly committed by males. While this violence may represent a small percentage of men, it is nevertheless quite troubling. Our society could be radically changed if men were more secure with their masculinity and were more caring and compassionate.

Compassion Needs to be Cultivated

We humans have a great capacity for compassion, but it's a not always in the forefront of our consciousness. More often, we are on autopilot focused on just trying to get through the day, fighting traffic, answering e-mails, working to-do lists, and getting to classes and meetings on time. Let's face it; compassion does not come naturally, especially in a culture that measures self- worth on the basis of narcissistic values like social status, financial or political power.

Cultivating compassion requires a quality of mindfulness that comes only from intentional practice and reflection. Meditation is just one way to enhance one's capacity for compassion.

The Healthy Brain

We cannot possibly know anything about human health and well-being without understanding something about the brain. The brain is thought be one of the most complex structures in the known universe. Although it only weighs about 3 pounds, the brain is made up of 100 billion cells (neurons) that interact with thousands of other neurons to make up as many as 100 trillion neural connections (Hanson, 2011).

We can think of the brain as the human command and control center somewhat like the central processing unit in a computer. Interacting with other parts of our body, the brain plays a pivotal role in virtually everything that makes us human.

Neuroplasticity and the Brain

There has been much talk lately about the neuroplasticity of the brain. Much of it is from advertisers who are trying to capitalize on the relatively new discovery to profit from brain improvement potions or training schemes. But, the implications of the revolutionary discovery that the brain can generate new neurons (neurogenesis) far exceeds the self-serving motivations of profiteers. Sharon Begley (2008) reported that the discovery of neuroplasticity revealed the extraordinary potential to actually change our own brains for the better, in effect, to become better human beings. This is hopeful news at a time when our world is so full of violence, racial prejudice, and bigotry.

The discovery of neuroplasticity was an outgrowth of many scientific experiments that took place over several decades, with mice, birds, rats, primates, and eventually, humans. No one believed that neurogenesis was possible, primarily because as pointed out, Santiago Ramon Y Cajal, a highly respected Nobel prize-winning neuroscientist, asserted in 1913 that once the brain was full developed in childhood it was incapable of changing - it was "fixed, ended, and immutable" (Begley 2008, p. 5). Ramon Y Cajal was so respected that his thinking about the fixed nature of the brain remained dogma for almost a century until the determined and persistent work of researchers uncovered the truth about the brain's plastic nature.

One of those researchers was Fred "Rusty" Gage a neuroscientist with the Salk Institute (Begley, 2008). His discovery provided credence to the centuries-old claim of Buddhism, i.e., that meditation could help people become more kind and compassionate. At a meeting of the Mind and Life Institute, an organization devoted to understanding the science of human emotions for the betterment of humankind, Gage told His Holiness the Dalai Lama that the discovery of neuroplasticity meant that *"the environment and our experiences change our brain, so who you are as a person changes by virtue of the environment you live in and the experiences you have".*

Healthy Brains Make for a Healthy Society

Human health and well-being depend upon how well the differentiated parts of the brain work together as a system (Siegel, 2017): *How we regulate our emotions, thoughts, attention, behavior, and relationships is dependent on integrative fibers of the brain (p. 82).*

Medical science has affirmed that without healthy brains, a society cannot be healthy. Sadly, our society has not come to grips with this reality. Many children do not receive the nurturing attention they need to form healthy brain architecture. This is one conclusion of the *Center for the Developing Child at Harvard* (2017), that emphasizes the critical importance of providing the optimal conditions for a child's early brain development. They use the analogy of building a solid foundation in order to have a stable house. When the early construction of brain architecture is weakened either in utero or in the first few years of a child's life, the brain's various parts fail to successfully interconnect. Recall the words of Fred Gage, that our brains are sculpted by our environment and the everyday experiences of life. When children do not receive the loving care they need during the crucial window of brain development, they may suffer long-term difficulty regulating their emotions.

Besides the obvious effects that poorly wired brain architecture has on learning, the effects on the emotional lives of children can be even more far reaching. For example, approximately 40% of early deaths are due to emotional or behavioral causes (Schroeder, 2007). Many of these brain-based behavioral problems stem from an inability to control one's emotions due to compromised brain architecture that occurred during early childhood. The inability to control emotions has huge consequences for society.

Antidotes to Trauma and Toxic Stress

Fortunately, the experience of trauma during childhood does not automatically sentence someone to a lifetime of poor physical and mental health. Of course, the most important thing is to prevent child maltreatment before it occurs. This can be facilitated through parent training programs, public service announcements, educating the general public about the scourge of adverse childhood experiences, and including age appropriate curricula in middle and high schools. Childhood toxic stress can also be reduced considerably by addressing poverty that can negatively affect a child's brain development (Luby, 2013).

For children who have experienced maltreatment, there are several possible antidotes that can be helpful. Perhaps the most important of these is for children to have caring and loving adults in their lives. The Centers for Disease Control and Prevention (2014) uses the acronym of SSNR's to describe the critical qualities that children need the most from adults: SAFE, STABLE, and NURTURING relationships. Such relationships serve as an anchor in the lives of children by buffering stress and consistently providing the message that they are safe and loved. As Van der Kolk (2014) put it: "if you feel safe and loved, your brain becomes specialized in exploration, play, and cooperation. If you are frightened and unwanted, it specializes in managing feelings of fear and abandonment" (p. 56).

Because stress resides in the body, learning to gradually inhabit one's body through programs like yoga can be helpful in overcoming stress trauma. A study by Seppalla et al. (2014) found that a breathing-based yoga resulted in reduced PTSD symptoms such as anxiety, and respiration rates in Afghanistan or Iraq veterans. Nadine Burke Harris (2018), a pediatrician and leading expert in childhood trauma, provides the following formula for ameliorating the effects of ACES: mental health treatment, healthy relationships, exercise, nutrition, sleep and meditation.

According to a review of mindfulness-based studies for children conducted by the departments of Internal Medicine and Pediatrics at Johns Hopkins Hospital (Ortiz & Sibinga, 2017), high-quality, structured instruction in mindfulness may also mitigate the effects of stress and trauma related to childhood adversity.

Understanding how the brain develops and is affected by both positive and negative forces, especially during a child's early development, provides an important window into how we can provide optimal conditions for healthy brain development. Safe, consistent, and nurturing human relationships along with mindfulness-based interventions are providing encouraging prospects for primary prevention programs.

Chapter Summary

- ✓ To flourish is "to grow or develop in a healthy or vigorous way, especially as the result of a particularly favorable environment".
- ✓ Contemplation refers to a variety of ways in which people explore their inner lives through reflection, introspection, and meditation.
- ✓ Mindfulness is to be aware and to live awake in the present moment.
- ✓ During meditation, it is normal for your mind to wander. Breathing, drifting away, and gently coming back is all a part of the process of meditation.
- ✓ The mistreatment of children during the critical years of brain development, may be one of society's greatest unaddressed public health problems.
- ✓ The human brain is responsible for virtually everything that makes us human such as: emotions, movement, communication, and keeping us safe via the fight or flight response.
- ✓ To empathize is to almost experience the same feeling of another individual as if you were in that person's shoes. Compassion is a desire to relieve someone else's suffering.

Chapter Review Questions

1) What is the difference between intrinsic and extrinsic values?
2) What is "positive psychology"?
3) True or False? When your mind wanders during meditation it means you are doing something wrong.
4) What is "mindfulness"?
5) What is the difference between empathy and compassion?
6) What did the section on Healthy Brains cite as one of the greatest unaddressed public health problems?
7) Can meditation increase compassion? If so, how?
8) The Harvard Study of Adult Development resulted in four major lessons of happiness. What were they?

References

4 lessons from the longest-running study on happiness. (2017, April 13). Retrieved from **https://ideas.ted.com/4-lessons-from-the-longest-running-study-on-happiness/**

Apostle, H.G. & Gerson, L.P. (1991). *Aristotle: Selected works*. Peripatetic Press.

Armstrong, K. (2011). *Twelve steps to a compassionate life.* AnchorBooks.

Barbezat, D., & Bush, M. (2014). *Contemplative practices in higher education: Powerful methods to transform teaching and learning.* Jossey-Bass, a Wiley brand.

Begley, S. (2008). *Train your mind, change your brain: How a new science reveals our extraordinary potential to transform ourselves.* Ballantine Books.

Black, D. S., & Fernando, R. (2013). Mindfulness Training and Classroom Behavior Among Lower-Income and Ethnic Minority Elementary School Children. *Journal of Child and Family Studies, 23*(7), 1242-1246. doi:10.1007/s10826-013-9784-4

Burke Harris, N. (2018). *The deepest well: Healing the long-term effects of childhood adversity*. Houghton Mifflin.

Can Meditation Lead to Lasting Change? (n.d.). Retrieved from **https://greatergood.berkeley.edu/article/item/can_meditation_lead_to_lasting_change**

Center on the Developing Child at Harvard University. (n.d.). Retrieved from **https://developingchild.harvard.edu/**

Center for Disease Control (2014). Essentials for Childhood: Safe, stable, nurturing relationships and environments. **www.cdc.gov/violenceprevention/pdf/essentials_for_childhood_framework.pdf**

Condon, P., Desbordes, G., Miller, W. B., & Desteno, D. (2013). Meditation Increases Compassionate Responses to Suffering. *Psychological Science, 24*(10), 2125-2127.

Crompton, T. (2010). *Common Cause: The case for working with our cultural values.* Oxfam GB. .**https://policy-practice.oxfam.org.uk/publications/common-cause-the-case-for-working-with-our-cultural-values-112367**

Crowley, M. J., Nicholls, S. S., Mccarthy, D., Greatorex, K., Wu, J., & Mayes, L. C. (2017, 03). Innovations in practice: Group mindfulness for adolescent anxiety - results of an open trial. *Child and Adolescent Mental Health.*

Felitti, V.J., et al., (1998). Relationship of childhood abuse and household dysfunction to many of the leading causes of death in adults: the adverse childhood experiences (ACE) study. *American Journal of Preventative Medicine, 14*, 245-258.

Flynn, R., & Kelly, B. (1986). *Our town, by Thornton Wilder.*

Galante, J., Bekkers, M., Mitchell, C., & Gallacher, J. (2016). Loving-Kindness Meditation Effects on Well-Being and Altruism: A Mixed-Methods Online RCT. *Applied Psychology: Health and Well-Being, 8*(3), 322-350.

Goleman, D. D. (2017). *Altered Traits Science Reveals How Meditation Changes Your Mind, Brain, and Body.* Avery Pub Group.

Hanson, R. (2011). *Buddha's brain: The practical neuroscience of happiness, love, and wisdom.* Readhowyouwant.com.

Kabat-Zinn, J. (2005). *Coming to our senses: Healing ourselves and the world through mindfulness.* Hyperion.

Kabat-Zinn, J. (2006). Mindfulness-Based Interventions in Context: Past, Present, and Future. *Clinical Psychology: Science and Practice, 10*(2), 144-156.

Kabat-Zinn, J. (2014). *Wherever you go, there you are mindfulness meditation in everyday life.* Hachette Books.

Kennedy, R. F. (2014, September 15). *Robert F. Kennedy on GDP.* Retrieved from **https://www.youtube.com/watch?v=t6U2irFSYHo**

Lama, D. (2011). *Beyond religion: Ethics for a whole world.* Houghton Mifflin Harcourt.

Lopez, S.J., Pedrotti, J.T., & Snyder, C.R. (2015*). Positive psychology: The scientific and practical exploration of human strengths.* Sage.

Luby, M. J. (2013). *Effects of Poverty on Childhood Brain Development.* Retrieved from **https://jamanetwork.com/journals/jamapediatrics/fullarticle/1761544**

Marx, J. (2004). *Season of life: A football star, a boy, a journey to manhood*. Simon & Schuster.

Maslow, A. H. (1971). *The farther reaches of human nature.* Viking.

Medina, C. C. (2015, April 27). *Breakthrough Magnet School Chosen the Best in America.* Retrieved from **http://www.courant.com/community/hc-ugc-article-breakthrough-magnet-school-chosen-the-best-i-2015-04-27-story.html**

Mosher, D. L. & Tomkins, S.S. (1988). Scripting the macho man: Hypermasculine socialization. The Journal of Sex Research, 25(1), 60-84.

Myrdal, G. (1944). *The American dilemma: The Negro problem and American democracy*. Harper.

Norden, J. (2007). *Understanding the brain.* Teaching Company.

Ortiz, R., & Sibinga, E. (2017). The Role of Mindfulness in Reducing the Adverse Effects of Childhood Stress and Trauma. *Children, 4*(3), 16.

Palmer, P. J. (2014). *Healing the Heart of Democracy: The Courage to Create a Politics Worthy of.* John Wiley & Sons.

Peterson, C., & Seligman, M. E. (2004). *Character strengths and virtues: A handbook and classification.* Oxford University Press.

Powell, A., Feldscher, K, Mineo, L., Walsh, C. &. Rowling, J. K. (2017). *Over nearly 80 years, Harvard study has been showing how to live a healthy and happy life.* Retrieved **from https://news.harvard.edu/gazette/story/2017/04/over-nearly-80-years-harvard-study-has-been-showing-how-to-live-a-healthy-and-happy-life/**

Powell, A., Sniffin-Marinoff, M., Walsh, C., & Mineo, L. (2010, November 11). *Wandering mind not a happy mind.* Retrieved from **https://news.harvard.edu/gazette/story/2010/11/wandering-mind-not-a-happy-mind/**

Rogers, C. (1961). *On becoming a person: A therapist's view of psychotherapy.* Houghton Mifflin

Rosenberg, L. (1998). *Breath by breath: The liberating practice of insight meditation.* Shambhala.

Sapolsky, R. M. (2017). *Behave: The biology of humans at our best and worst.* Penguin Press.

Schroeder, S. A. (2007). We Can Do Better — Improving the Health of the American People. *New England Journal of Medicine, 357*(12), 1221-1228.

Seppälä, E. M., Nitschke, J. B., Tudorascu, D. L., Hayes, A., Goldstein, M. R., Nguyen, D. T., & Davidson, R. J. (2014). Breathing-Based Meditation Decreases Posttraumatic Stress Disorder Symptoms in U.S. Military Veterans: A Randomized Controlled Longitudinal Study. *Journal of Traumatic Stress, 27*(4), 397-405.

Seppälä, E. M. (2013). 20 Scientific reasons to start meditating today. Retrieved from:
https://www.psychologytoday.com/us/blog/feeling-it/201309/20-scientific-reasons-start-meditating-today

Sibinga, E. M., Webb, L., Ghazarian, S. R., & Ellen, J. M. (2015, 12). School-Based Mindfulness Instruction: An RCT. *Pediatrics, 137*(1). doi:10.1542/peds.2015-2532

Siegel, D. J. (2011). *Mindsight: The new science of personal transformation.* Bantam Books.

Siegel, D. J. (2017). *Mind: A journey to the heart of being human.* W W Norton & Co.

Snyder, C. R., Lopez, S. J., & Pedrotti, J. T. (2015). *Positive psychology: The scientific and practical explorations of human strengths.* SAGE.

Thoreau, H. D., & Emerson, R. W. (1995). *Walden*. Thoreau. Dent.

Van Der Kolk, B. (2014). *The body keeps the score: Brain, mind, and body in the healing of trauma.* Penguin Books. (2016).

Weng, H. Y., Fox, A. S., Shackman, A. J., Stodola, D. E., Caldwell, J. Z., Olson, M. C., Davidson, R. J. (2013). Compassion Training Alters Altruism and Neural Responses to Suffering. *Psychological Science, 24*(7), 1171-1180.

Chapter 6

Social and Emotional Learning

By Carol Ciotto, MS and Matthew Martin, PhD

Chapter Objectives

After reading this chapter, students should be able to:

- ✓ Understand the social and emotional competencies associated with intra- and inter-personal success;
- ✓ Discuss opportunities for direct application of these competencies to both academic and personal life; and
- ✓ Recognize the skills and resources needed to be a successful college student.

Social and Emotional Learning

"When our emotional health is in a bad state, so is our level of self-esteem. We have to slow down and deal with what is troubling us, so that we can enjoy the simple joy of being happy and at peace with ourselves." -Jess C. Scott

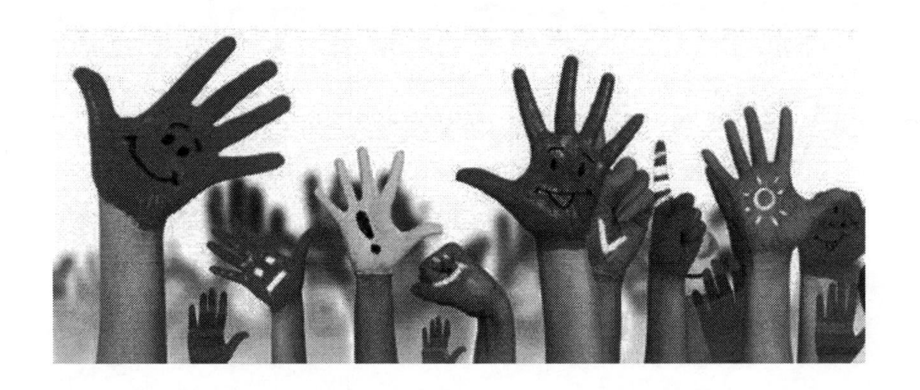

What is Social Emotional Learning (SEL)?

Social emotional learning (SEL) provides a framework that allows individuals the ability to recognize, manage, and express the social and emotional aspects of their lives to successfully accomplish a variety of tasks such as learning, developing relationships, solving problems, setting goals, and expressing compassion for self and others.

Research shows that the development of positive social and emotional skills can have a direct impact on one's behavior, learning, career, and overall health and well-being. Continued practice and nurturing of one's social and emotional well-being allows individuals to realize their potential, deal with the ongoing stresses of attending college and successfully graduate, have steady employment, and be a positive and productive contributing member of their community (Jones, Greenberg, & Crowley, 2015).

Strong SEL skills are linked to:

- ✓ higher academic performance
- ✓ increased productivity at work
- ✓ decreased emotional distress
- ✓ decreased stress and depression
- ✓ improved attitudes toward self, school, work and others.

The Benefits of Social Emotional Learning (SEL)

The goal of developing SEL is to address social and emotional needs that help people be successful during their academic endeavors, in their professional career and in other life pursuits. In particular, one must be able to control their emotions, work collaboratively and communicate effectively with others, and make sound choices about personal and social decisions (Yoder, 2013).

Researchers have found that interventions to improve SEL skills have led to positive results in school, work, and in the community for participants who were in their twenties. Specifically, Hawkins and his colleagues (2008) found that many of the participants had graduated college, had higher household incomes and more community involvement than the individuals in the control group. Also, the study participants had fewer symptoms of mental health disorders (Hawkins, Kosterman, Catalano, Hill & Abbott, 2008).

In addition to emotional and academic benefits of SEL, many employers are looking for individuals with highly developed social-emotional skills who are effective critical thinkers, problem solvers, and team players who have the ability to collaborate and communicate with people from diverse backgrounds. Furthermore, possessing these skills has been shown to improve college graduates' employability and future earnings (Goleman, 1995). For example, according to the National Association of Colleges and Employers (2015), SEL skills are one of the main factors that employers consider when interviewing applicants, which often sets candidates apart who have similar academic records. It also improves educational outcomes and has monetary benefits (Table 1).

Table 1. Academic and Economical Benefits of SEL Skills

	Percentage Advantage per SEL Student	**Monetary Benefit Per Student**
More/better/higher...		
High school graduation rates	6%	$367,687
College attendance	11	$637,621
College degrees	11	$1,138,054
Less/fewer/lower....		
High school dropouts	7.5-26%	
STD diagnosis	39	$ 9,940
Arrests	19	$175,702
Any clinical mental health disorder	13.5	
Diagnosis of conduct disorder	10	$3,950,000

SEL CORE COMPETENCIES

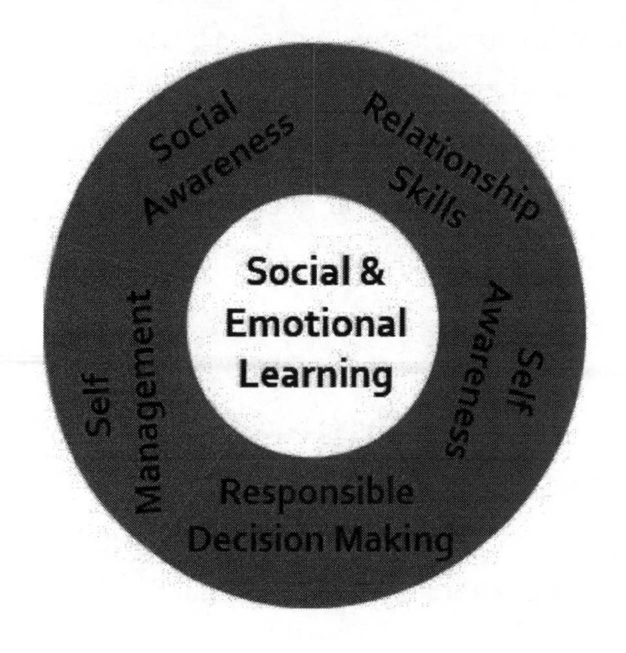

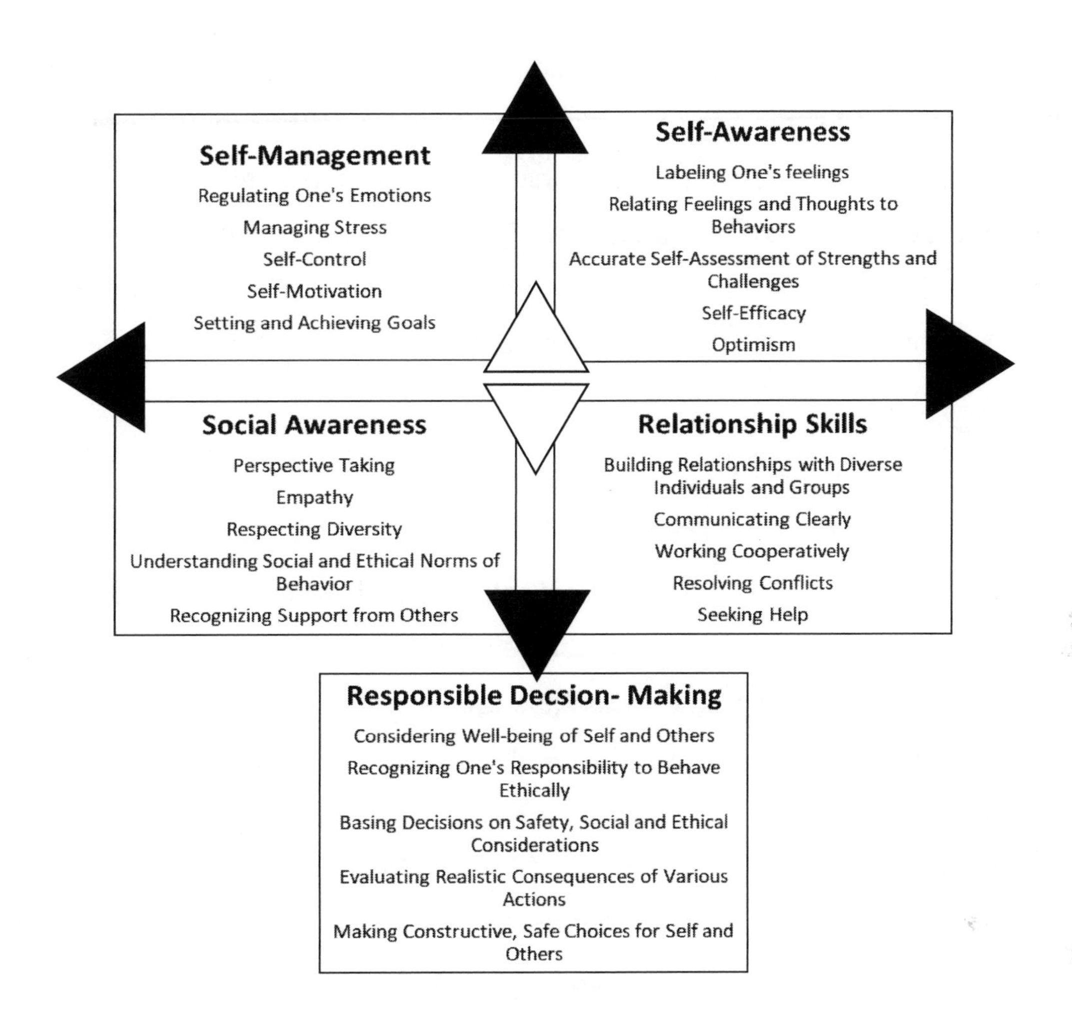

Five Core Competencies of SEL

SEL includes five core competencies that address the essential skills needed for college students to be successful in school and to be ready to pursue a career in their field of interest. The five competencies of SEL are (CASEL, 2017):

1) Self-Awareness,
2) Self-Management,
3) Responsible Decision-Making,
4) Relationship Management and
5) Social Awareness

The Collaborative for Academic, Social, and Emotional Learning (CASEL) integrated framework can be used to help individuals increase SEL competencies with regards to building relationships and communicating with others, as well as developing an awareness of how one's actions and decisions affect those around them. As one masters these competencies, they begin to develop concern for others, make good choices, and take responsibility for their behaviors.

Self-Awareness

Self-awareness involves the ability to identify, describe and understand one's thoughts and emotions and the potential impact they may have on one's behavior. This consists of accurately evaluating one's strengths and limitations and having a well-grounded sense of self-efficacy and confidence. Individuals who have a strong sense of their own strengths and weaknesses often make positive life choices and persist when engaged in challenging tasks (Ryan, Gheen, & Midgley, 1998; Zimmerman, 2000). For example, do you actively seek out assistance from your professors when struggling with course content or assignments? Or do you tend to procrastinate and not seek help from others?

Success in college can be achieved when you reflect about and actively work on improving your interpersonal and social skills. For example, when working on a group assignment/project, you must understand what your responsibilities are and how you will need to communicate with your peers in order to organize and develop a plan for accomplishing the group task. It is also important to recognize your own capabilities and work habits, so you can better communicate with your group how you can best contribute to the assignment.

High level of self-awareness is the ability to recognize how your thoughts, feelings, and actions are interconnected. Specifically, self-awareness is an ongoing evaluative process of inwardly focusing on your actions and the actions and feedback of others (social comparison) to gain a greater understanding of self. This evaluative process allows you to consider alternatives to complete a task, solve problems and make progress toward meeting individual goals. Dr. Merriman from the University of Georgia described the self-aware adult as one who:

- ✓ Can direct their own learning.
- ✓ Can draw on past experiences to make decisions
- ✓ Is problem-centered and is interested in applying what they have learned in a timely manner.
- ✓ Is internally motivated to learn.

Without self-awareness, our decision-making and thinking can be influenced by self-deception which is a thought process that makes communication with others difficult and impedes the learning process particularly when working in groups. Furthermore, if you do not actively work on developing self-awareness skills, it is difficult to learn about ourselves, further develop our strengths and be aware of our weaknesses. The more effective we can evaluate our strengths and weaknesses and critically reflect about how we are acting, the more control we have over events in our lives (Steiner, 2014). Try Activity #1 and #2 to learn more about yourself.

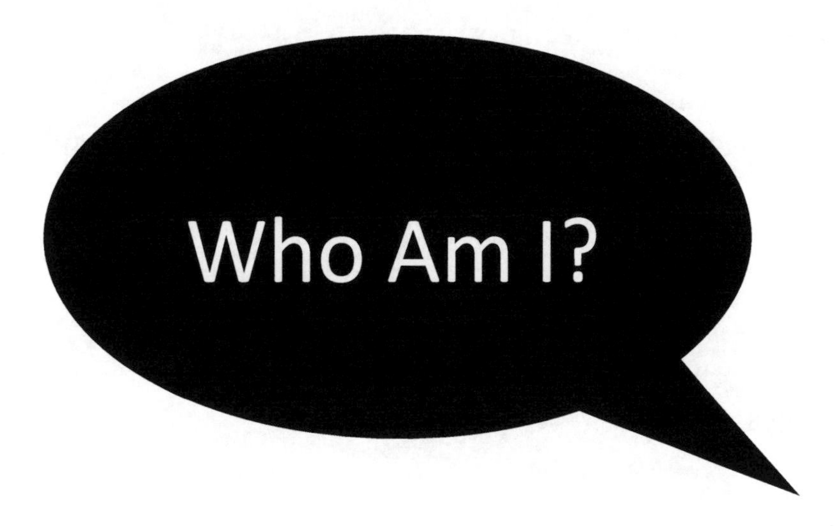

Activity #1: Creating My Personal Story

- ✓ Tell "your personal story" by drawing yourself in the middle of a large sheet of paper.
- ✓ Around this figure, make notes about significant role models, personal experiences, and other meaningful events that have impacted your life.
- ✓ Next, draw figures of those individuals that have made a difference in your life by shaping your values and belief system. These could be parents, grandparents, siblings, other relatives, friends, mentors, teachers, etc.
- ✓ Reflect on this story.

Activity #2: "Mirror, Mirror, on the Wall".

Diversity includes, but is not limited to, race, religion, ethnicity, gender, sexual orientation, age, physical and mental ability, language, nation of origin, etc. Answer the questions below; if you are comfortable, share your answers with someone you don't know in the class.

1) When I look in the mirror, I see:

2) If I had to describe myself in four words, I would say that I am a:

   ____________________ ____________________

   ____________________ ____________________

3) One experience that I have had that helped me to form this description of myself was:

Self-Management

Self-management is the ability to effectively control one's thoughts, emotions, and behaviors in varied and/or challenging situations. This includes stress management, impulse control, organizational skills, self-discipline, self-motivation, and the ability to meet personal and academic goals (CASEL 2017).

Well-developed self-management skills also helps you be successful while you are in college, in your career and throughout your life. These skills include setting goals, managing your time, staying motivated, and concentrating on personal and work-related tasks.

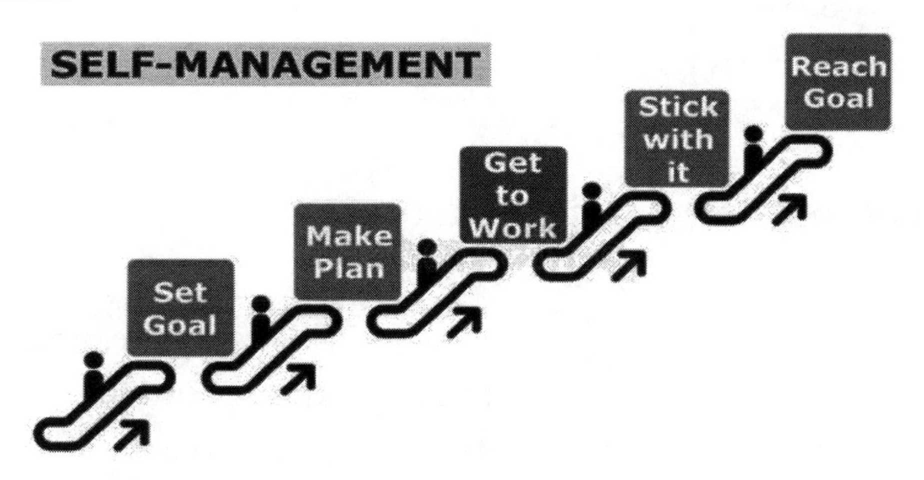

As the self-management figure above illustrates, after setting a goal, it is important that you develop a structured action plan which includes specific steps/actions to meet your goal. For instance, a second-year college student wants to increase his G.P.A. from (2.50 to 3.00) next semester. To achieve this goal, the following steps could be included in his plan: a) study at the library three days per week; b) seek out campus math and science tutors; (c) meet with my professors at least once a month to discuss academic progress; and (d) participate in study groups prior to exams. This example plan helps one monitor progress towards meeting the goal and gives tangible things to actively achieve it.

Activity #3: Career Aspirations

- ✓ **Setting the Goal:** Write one career-related goal that you hope to accomplish upon graduation.

  Career Goal:

- ✓ **Challenge(s) to Meet Goal:** Identify two obstacles that might prevent you from meeting your career goal.

  Obstacle One:

  Obstacle Two

- ✓ **Action Plan:** Describe two strategies that you can implement to overcome the obstacles you have identified.

  Strategy #1:

  Strategy #2:

Responsible Decision Making

Responsible decision-making involves learning how to make appropriate and respectful choices about personal behavior and social interactions based on the consideration of ethical standards, safety concerns, social norms and the well-being of self and others. This competency includes the capacity to identify problems and develop appropriate solutions to social, emotional or cognitive challenges (Payton et al., 2000).

The following steps can be used to make responsible decisions: (a) describe the situation in writing or verbally if a decision needs to be made quickly; (b) list in writing or out loud to yourself the possible decisions; (c) share the list with a trusted friend, family member or another important person in your life; (d) listen and consider their feedback; (e) decide which decision you are most comfortable with based on your own reflection and the feedback from others; and (f) act on your decision and evaluate the results (Meeks, Heit & Page, 2013).

Sometimes we make quick decisions without taking the time to consider different options (impulse decisions). Other times we consider our options and make positive life choices (controlled decisions; See Activity #3)

Activity #3: My Choices

Source: adapted from **http://www.umassd.edu/fycm/decisionmaking/collegechoices/**

1) As you read the questions, check the box that most closely applies to you right now; either impulse problem or controlling impulse.
2) On a scale from 1 to 10, with 10 being the highest, how would you rate your decision-making abilities based on your responses below?
3) What's your plan for either continuing to make good decisions or making better decisions?

MOVING AWAY FROM YOUR GOALS IMPULSE PROBLEMS	MOVING TOWARDS YOUR GOALS CONTROLLING IMPULSES
1) Who are your friends? Do they get you closer or further away from your goals?	
Hanging with others who have limited to no college goals	Hanging with others who have realistic college goals
2) Do your friends get drunk often?	
Hanging with others who have substance control problems	Hanging with others who can say no to substances
3) How serious are your friends about graduating?	
Hanging with others who have academic problems	Hanging with good students
4) Are you making responsible decisions about attending classes?	
Skip classes	Go to every class
5) Are you making responsible decisions about doing your homework?	
Not doing homework – it doesn't matter	Giving homework your best – It matters; learning builds sequentially through studying and completing assignments
6) Are you making responsible decisions about saying "No"	
Having trouble saying "no" to bad choices	Learning to say "no" to bad choices even if it is hard; others may be disappointed, gets better over time
7) Are you making responsible decisions about drinking?	

<table>
<tr><td>Getting drunk, Thursday through Sunday – a dangerous trend, bad for academics, your health, and higher chance of making other bad decisions while intoxicated</td><td>Drinking, or not, but not getting drunk; having fun without getting drunk</td></tr>
<tr><td colspan="2">8) Are you making responsible decisions about use of substances?</td></tr>
<tr><td>Messing with substances
They're illegal. What are the consequences if caught?</td><td>Saying "no" to offers of substances</td></tr>
<tr><td colspan="2">9) Are you making responsible decisions about gambling?</td></tr>
<tr><td>Becoming a real problem. Can create tremendous problems with debt</td><td>Not gambling with money</td></tr>
<tr><td colspan="2">10) Are you making responsible decisions about controlling impulses</td></tr>
<tr><td>Real trouble controlling impulses
Doing what you "feel" like rather than thinking through the consequences results in a lot of trouble</td><td>Counting to "10" strategies - learning to put the brakes on impulses - don't make immediate decisions around risky choices</td></tr>
<tr><td colspan="2">11) Are you making responsible decisions about controlling anger?</td></tr>
<tr><td>Physical fights to solve anger
College is about increasingly learning to use your brain to solve problems</td><td>Using words to solve anger</td></tr>
<tr><td colspan="2">12) Are you making responsible decisions about getting involved on campus?</td></tr>
<tr><td>Not participating in any clubs, groups, service learning programs, intramurals, etc.</td><td>Getting involved is a great way to forget about your own troubles and help you to stay focused</td></tr>
<tr><td colspan="2">13) Are you making responsible decisions about your academic integrity?</td></tr>
<tr><td>Lying, cheating, and copying; it's all trouble and can get you dismissed</td><td>Honesty is the best policy
What would your "mother" say?</td></tr>
<tr><td colspan="2">14) Are you making responsible decisions about weapons?</td></tr>
<tr><td>Weapons of any sort on/off campus;
"They're illegal but I won't get caught"</td><td>Saying no to these choices</td></tr>
<tr><td colspan="2">15) Are you making responsible decisions about taking self-responsibility?</td></tr>
<tr><td>Blaming others for your problems
'I've got problems because of my parents or my teachers"</td><td>In the end, you look in the mirror, and know the decisions and choices that you made are responsible for your successes and failures</td></tr>
</table>

Relationship Skills/Management

Relationship skills involve the ability to establish and maintain healthy and rewarding relationships with individuals and/or groups. This competency includes the ability to communicate clearly, be cooperative, be an active listener, avoid inappropriate social pressure, negotiate conflict, seek and/or offer help when necessary (CASEL, 2017).

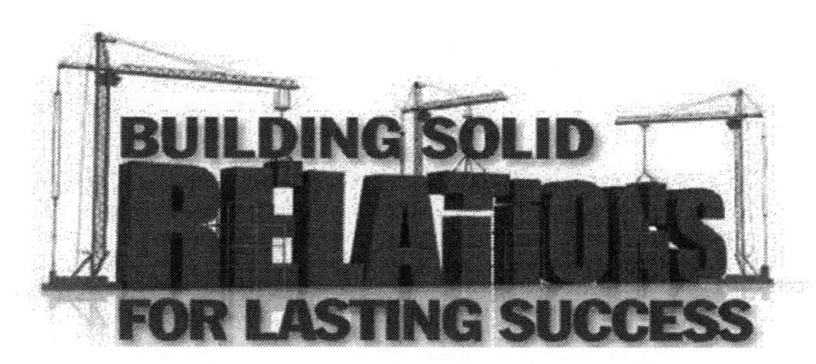

Individuals who enjoy building positive relationships experience higher levels of emotional well-being and have a stronger sense of self-confidence than those without positive peer relationships. Furthermore, relationship skills help students build healthy social networks which can reduce feelings of loneliness and increase social connectedness with other students and faculty (Dymnicki, Sambolt & Kidron, 2013). Researchers have also found that relationship skills that are well developed results in individuals who are self-confident, trusting, empathic, competent in communicating, and relate well with others (Cohen, Onunaku, Clothier & Poppe, 2005).

Some actions you can take to build a social network include: joining a student club, intramurals, a study group with peers, taking a fitness class through RECentral, or attending a campus event.

Activity #4: Roommate Scenarios

Discuss the scenarios in groups of 2-3 students.

Source: adapted from Renee Beason and Patrick Critzer (Radford University)

- ✓ Your roommate is disorganized and his or her stuff keeps reaching your side of the room.
- ✓ Your roommate has his or her significant other stay over every night.
- ✓ Your roommate talks loudly on the phone while you are studying.
- ✓ Your roommate frequently brings friends and alcohol into the room.
- ✓ Share another possible scenario with the group.

Social Awareness

Social awareness is the ability to embrace diversity by recognizing, understanding and appreciating the similarities and differences within and among individuals and groups. Being socially aware involves being accepting of different perspectives from individuals with diverse backgrounds and cultures with the hope that we can understand social and ethical norms for behavior. Social awareness is also the ability to identify and recognize emotions in other people to understand how those emotions influence particular social situations (Domitrovich, Durlak, Goren, & Weissberg, 2013).

Social awareness has also been described as: a) being aware of social injustices in your community or larger society; b) taking action and speaking out about social injustices; and c) promoting racial tolerance and respect which helps you function in an everchanging and diverse society (Green & Kamimura, 2003). In addition, Tsui's (2000) research on social awareness has shown that becoming more socially aware and being an advocate for social change helps create a more educated society and develops critical thinking skills.

As a starting point, stay informed about community issues on campus, in the community, state, and nation. Check out your university or community newspapers or quality media sources online or watch the news on television. Next, be an active participant in class discussions about current social issues and consider joining a student club or attending a rally at your university or local community that supports social justice issues that you are passionate about.

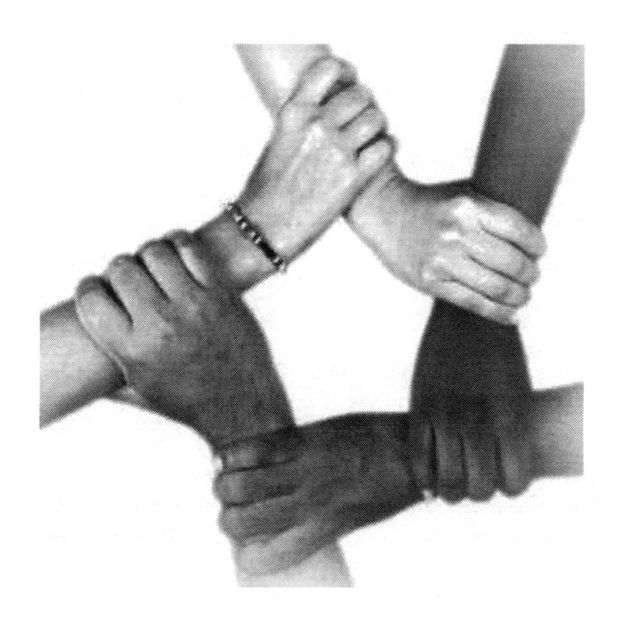

Activity #5: Improve your Social Awareness

Review the following eight steps; identify the ones you are doing well and the ones you can improve upon. For those that you can improve upon, brainstorm some strategies to improve your social awareness.

1) Learn to identify which types of situations make you uncomfortable, and then alter your behavior to make the best of your circumstances.
2) Learn to become aware of behaviors in other people that may cause you to respond negatively. As you are unlikely to be able to change the other person, you must be able to modify your own behavior to turn the situation into a positive experience.
3) Take ownership for your behavior and be willing to apologize for lapses or errors in judgment or insensitive actions.
4) Ask others for their honest feedback about the way you interact with them. Accept the negative feedback along with the positive (without getting defensive) and make changes accordingly.
5) Be aware of your body language. Non-verbal communication is more important than what you have to say. Positive body language will benefit your interactions with other people.
6) Learn to listen with genuine interest. Fight the urge to respond immediately and really listen to what the other person is trying to say.
7) Accept that improving your social skills is not an overnight process. Trying to improve or change too many things at once will be counterproductive as you will feel so uncomfortable that you may suffer an emotional hijacking.
8) Maximize your positive personality traits and use them to your advantage when interacting with others.

Source: **https://www.linkedin.com/pulse/8-steps-improve-your-social-awareness-bob-woodcock-mba/**

Developing SEL Through Physical Activity

"the brain and peripheral nervous system, the endocrine and immune systems, and indeed, all the organs of our body and all the emotional responses we have, share a common chemical language and are constantly communicating with one another."

- Dr. James Gordon (founder of the Center for Mind-Body Medicine)

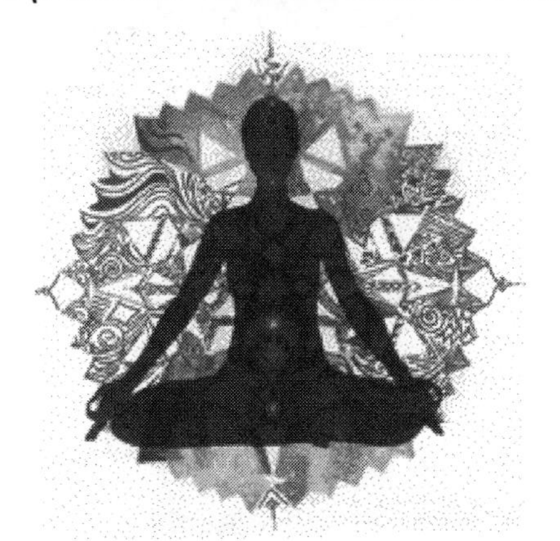

SEL enhances an individual's capacity to integrate skills, attitudes, and behaviors to effectively and properly handle daily tasks and challenges. Engaging in physical activity is a great way to develop these skills and contribute to ones' social and emotional development, cognition and overall fitness. We must first understand the important connection between the mind and body. Our thoughts, feelings, beliefs, and attitudes can have a direct impact on our body, which can ultimately affect our health (Hart, 2018)

Staying active is one of the best ways to keep our minds and bodies fit and healthy while improving our overall well-being and quality of life. Incorporating physical activity throughout your day can help you feel better, look better and live better. Most people notice they feel better over time as physical activity becomes a regular part of their lives.

Sitting uses far less energy than if we were to stand and or be actively moving. Studies show that sitting for long periods of time is very bad for your health and increases your risks of all kinds of dangerous diseases, especially later in life, such as high blood pressure, diabetes, obesity, and high cholesterol levels. Excessive sitting for extended periods of time can also increase the risk of death from cardiovascular disease and cancer. Engaging in even small bouts of physical activity or Brain Breaks (quick 1 - 2-minute activities that are fun, make you laugh and challenge your brain) throughout the day during extended periods of sitting can enhance the development of a host of positive effects (listed below) on ones' physical, social, emotional and cognitive development in several ways, especially as you age. (Laskowski, 2018).

Social & Emotional Benefits of Physical Activity:

- Makes you feel better and happier
- Fosters your sense of self-worth and makes you feel strong and powerful
- Can make you feel better about your appearance and, by meeting even small exercise goals, you'll feel a sense of achievement
- Reduces both anxiety and depression
- Raises levels of serotonin, endorphins and other chemicals that have a calming, anti-depressive effect
- Can help you to sleep better and may give you more energy
- Increases endorphins that boost your mood and can also boost your concentration skills
- Provides opportunities for self-expression
- Can make you feel more alert and may raise your self-esteem
- Can help you focus more clearly on your relationships, your job or your schoolwork, which may add to your feelings of self-confidence
- Improves attention span, memory, and learning
- Reduces stress and the effects of attention-deficit hyperactivity disorder
- Can help you cope in a healthy way, instead of resorting to negative behaviors
- Can help boost your immune system and reduce the impact of stress
- Boosts energy and brain power

As your emotional health and self-esteem improves, your social relations may also improve, and you may be more likely to reach out to others due to your increased self-confidence. Meeting others may be the first step toward building new relationships and developing a support network that can foster your social and emotional growth and development. We know the health-related benefits associated with being physically active, and now we can add SEL and brain power to that list.

For some quick physical activity/brain breaks that can help get you up and moving when you need a little boost, visit:

www.energizingbrainbreaks.com

Activity #4: Toe Tapping Brain Break

1) Stand Up.
2) Face your partner.
3) Both you and your partner put out your right leg and tap your right feet together 1 time and say "1" out loud.
4) Tap your left feet together 3 times and say "3" out loud.
5) Tap your right feet together 2 times and say "2" out loud.
6) Continue the 1, 3, 2 toe tapping pattern alternating feet.
7) See how fast you can go.

Chapter Summary

- ✓ According to Collaborative for Academic, Social, and Emotional Learning (CASEL), social and emotional learning is the process of developing students' and adults' social and emotional competencies--the knowledge, skills, attitudes, and behaviors that individuals need to make successful choices. SEL helps make individuals understand and regulate their emotions, successfully complete goals, take others' perspective or point of view, develop positive relationships, and make responsible decisions.
- ✓ Developing SEL skills improves student capacity to engage in academic learning and prepares students to meet college and career readiness standards. In order to participate in rigorous standards, students need to be able to regulate their emotions when they become frustrated, collaborate with their peers, communicate their ideas, and take the perspective of others.
- ✓ CASEL identifies five social and emotional competencies, which are composed of multiple skills and abilities:
  1) Self-awareness is the ability to recognize one's own feelings, interests, strengths, and limitations
  2) Self-management refers to when individuals regulate emotions and manage daily stressors
  3) Social awareness refers to perspective taking and to appreciate similarities and differences
  4) Relationship skills are when individuals exhibit prosocial behavior and demonstrate positive social skills in order to develop meaningful relationships
  5) Responsible decision making refers to when individuals make ethical decisions, and strengthen the ability to develop appropriate solutions to identified problems
- ✓ Research demonstrates that when students participate in activities that focus on these competencies, student prosocial behavior improves, students decrease in their participation of negative behaviors, and students improve in their academic achievement and overall success in life.

Chapter Review Questions

1) What is social and emotional learning (SEL)?
2) Identify and briefly describe the five core competencies of social and emotional learning?
3) How does the development of these core competencies impact us in school, career and in life?
4) The goal of social and emotional learning is to foster “knowledgeable, responsible, and caring” individuals. Why do you think these attributes are important? How do these attributes contribute to the development of a "well-rounded" individual and how will they help you to be successful in school, work, and life?
5) What are some examples of how social and emotional skills can contribute to success in various settings?
6) Provide an example of a behavioral change one might make to help them improve in each of the core competency skills?
7) Identify some key characteristics of a well-developed social-emotional individual.
8) What is meant by the brain -body connection and why is it important with regards to our overall health?
9) What are Brain Breaks and why are they important?
10) What role does physical activity play in the development of social emotional skills?

References

Adams, D. N., & Hamm, M. E. (1990). *Cooperative learning - Critical thinking and collaboration across the curriculum*. Springfield, IL: Charles C Thomas.

Clearly, T. J., & Zimmerman, B. J. (2004). Self-Regulation Empowerment Program: A school-based program to enhance self-regulated and self-motivated cycles of student learning. *Psychology in the Schools*, *41*, 537–550.

Cohen, J., Onunaku, N., Clothier, S., & Poppe, J. (2005). *Helping Young Children Succeed: Strategies to Promote Early Childhood Social and Emotional Development.* Washington, DC: National Conference of State Legislatures.

Collaborative for Academic, Social, and Emotional Learning (CASEL, 2017) Retrieved from **www.casel.org**

Denham, S. A., & Almeida, M. C. (1987). Children's social problem-solving skills, behavioral adjustment, and interventions: A meta-analysis evaluating theory and practice. *Journal of Applied Developmental Psychology, 8*, 391–409.

Domitrovich. C., Durlak, J., Goren, P., & Weissberg, R. (2013). *Effective social and emotional learning programs: Preschool and elementary school edition*. 2013 CASEL guide.

Durlak, J. A., Weissberg, R. P., Dymnicki, A. B., Taylor, R. D., & Schellinger, K. B. (2011). The impact of enhancing students' social and emotional learning: A meta-analysis of school-based universal interventions. *Child Development, 82*, 405-432

Dymnicki, A., Sambolt, M. & Kidron, Y. (2013). Improving, college and career readiness by incorporating social and emotional learning. *College & Career Readiness & Success Center at American Institutes for Research*, 1-23.

Galinsky, E. (2010). *Mind in the making*. New York, NY: Harper Collins.

Goleman, D. P. (1995). *Emotional Intelligence: Why It Can Matter More Than IQ for Character, Health and Lifelong Achievement*. Bantam Books, New York.

Greenberg, M., Weissberg, R., O'Brien, M., Zins, J., Fredericks, L., Resnik, H., et al. (2003). Enhancing school-based prevention and youth development through coordinated social, emotional, and academic learning. *American Psychologist, 58*(6/7), 466-474.

Gross, J. J. (2002). Emotional regulation: Affective, cognitive, and social consequences. *Psychophysiology*, *39*, 281–291.

Hawkins, J. D., Kosterman, R., Catalano, R. F., Hill, K. G., & Abbott, R. D. (2008). Effects of social development intervention in childhood 15 years later. *Archives of Pediatrics and Adolescent Medicine, 162*(12), 1133-1141.

Jones, D. E., Greenberg, M., & Crowley, M. (2015). Early social-emotional functioning and public health: The relationship between kindergarten social competence and future wellness. American Journal of Public Health, 105(11), 2283–90. Retrieved from **www.cfchildren.org/Portals/1/SS_Multi/ss_doc/early-social-emotional-functioning-and-public-health-AJPH-Jones-et-al-07-2015. Pdf**

Laskowski, E.R., What are the risks of sitting too much? (2018) Retrieved from **https://www.mayoclinic.org/healthy-lifestyle/adult-health/expert-answers/sitting/faq-20058005**

Meeks, L., Heit, P. & Page, R. (2013). Comprehensive School Health Education: Totally Awesome Strategies for Teaching Health

National Association of Colleges and Employers. (2014). Job Outlook 2015. Available from **www.naceweb.org**

Payton, J. W., Wardlaw, M. D., Graczyk, P. A., Bloodworth, M. R., Tompsett, C. J., & Weissberg, R. P. (2000). SEL: A framework for promoting mental health and reducing risk behavior in children and youth. *Journal of School Health, 70*(5), 179-185.

Romasz, T. E., Kantor, J. H., & Elias, M. (2004). Implementation and evaluation of urban school-based social-emotional learning programs. *Evaluation and Program Planning*, 27, 89–103.

Ryan, A., Gheen, M. H., & Midgley, C. (1998). Why do some students avoid asking for help? An examination of the interplay among students' academic efficacy, teachers' social-emotional role, and the classroom goal structure. *Journal of Educational Psychology*, *90*, 528–535

Steiner, P.F. (2014). The impact of the self-awareness process on learning and leading. *New England Journal of Higher Education*, 1-4.

Taylor, R. D., Oberle, E., Durlak, J. A. & Weissberg, R. P. (2017), Promoting Positive Youth Development through School-Based Social and Emotional Learning Interventions: A Meta-Analysis of Follow-Up Effects. *Child Development, 88*, 1156–1171.

Yoder, N. (2013). *Teaching the whole child: Instructional practices that support social and emotional learning in three teacher evaluation frameworks*. Washington, DC: American Institutes for Research Center on Great Teachers and Leaders.

Zimmerman, B.J. (2000). Self-efficacy: An essential motive to learn. *Contemporary Educational Psychology*, *25*, 82–91.

Chapter 7

Managing Stress for College Wellness

By Mike Voight, PhD, CMPC

Chapter Objectives

After reading this chapter, students should be able to:

- ✓ Compare the differences between stress, anxiety, and arousal;
- ✓ Describe the types of stressors and the impact of stress on individuals and society as a whole;
- ✓ Appraise and reflect upon the ability to cope with sources of stress;
- ✓ Analyze the different components of the A-B-C's of stress management;
- ✓ Identify contributing factors to the stress response (fight, flight, withdrawal, shock, tend and befriend);
- ✓ Explain physical, relaxation, and behavioral stress management techniques;
- ✓ Apply theoretical and practical concepts to one's own experiences to understand stress and its impact on health and our lives; and
- ✓ Integrate and practice stress management techniques into one's daily-weekly activities.

Defining Stress – ABC's of Stress Management

"A scientific concept which is too well known and too little understood."
- Hans Selye

Defining Stress

The quote above typifies the paradox involved in the study of stress and its impact on people's lives and on society as a whole. It is the aim of this chapter to improve your understanding of what stress is, the many sources of stress, as well as improving how you manage stress in your life.

Hans Selye, a pioneer in the study of stress, defined stress as the "nonspecific response of the body to any demand made upon it." Stress is perceived differently from one person to the next, and even if two people experience the same stressor, each person will have their own specific way of dealing, or not dealing with it. Some may perceive a stressor as a major blow, whereby another may perceive it as a minor annoyance. This is why this particular definition is cited here, as it covers all the bases. Anything that has the potential to cause us stress is referred to as a stressor, or a stimulus. These stressors could be from within, our own thoughts and feelings, or from an external source, such as something physical (i.e., something we touch that is hot), social (i.e., doing a class presentation or having to converse with those you do not know), or environmental (i.e., inclement weather).

There are typically two types of stressors: good stressors, referred to as eustress, and negative stressors, called distress. Eustress are the types of stressors that helps us perform better and become stronger, like the stress of physical conditioning and fitness. The more we stress our physical systems through increasing the resistance of weights or the increased intensity in our cardio workouts, the stronger the system will respond, and the healthier and more efficient our systems become. Without the stress of exams and grades, would you do your due diligence with the reading, homework, and studying to learn as much as you can in each of your classes?

Probably not, for the majority. Conversely, distress are stressors that are perceived as negative which have an adverse effect on how you think and feel emotionally and physically. Some stressors are acute (one-time, out-of-the-blue types), such as loud noises or receiving bad news, whereby others could be chronic, which are longer duration, such as mourning the death of a loved one. Common stressors experience by many college students are the daily hassles experienced, such as dealing with a roommate, the ever-present reading and studying that comes with college, as well as the daily worries around finances, and even fitting in with a peer group. Research has revealed that college students are challenged more by these daily hassles than major life events. The most common stressor for college students is lack of money.

Activity #1: Hassles and Reactions

Reflect on the daily hassles you experience and list them below. Across from each, what is the physical, emotional, or mental reaction to each. A sample is included below.

Daily Hassle	Reaction
i.e. Finding a parking spot on campus.	i.e. I get so frustrated! I fear I will be late for class.

Stress and Anxiety

Stress can sometimes be confused with anxiety and arousal. When a stressor is perceived as a threat to one's self esteem or in the rare occurrence, a physical threat, it produces extreme psychological and emotional reactions which could include anxiety, fear, frustration, anger, depression, or other negative emotional and mood states. Some confuse stress with one of these reactions, anxiety.

Anxiety is an unpleasant emotional response characterized by an overreaction to an expectation of a future threat or worry. Anxiety can result in excessive cognitive worrying and negative self-talk, which impacts one's confidence level.-This coincides with the belief that one will not be able to control one's thinking patterns and thus, cannot change the situation they are in. Arousal is the physiological reaction to worrying over a future stressor or threat, which is not guaranteed to occur. This is also referred to as somatic anxiety. Arousal is said to occur when there is muscle tension and bracing, shallow, rapid breathing, and behavioral pacing because of the anxious worrying. Anxiety can be experienced in the short term, or "state" and also across a longer term, referred to as "trait."

Long term exposure to stress and anxiety could lead to burnout. Burnout can occur when one believes they do have lost the control or resources to bring about change. According to Psychology Today,

> "Burnout is not a simple result of long hours. The cynicism, depression, and lethargy of burnout can occur when you're not in control of how you carry out your job, when you're working toward goals that don't resonate with you, and when you lack social support. If you don't tailor your responsibilities to match your true calling, or at least take a break once in a while, you could face a mountain of mental and physical health problems."

Fight or Flight Responses

In times of adversity, especially when one appraises a stressor as a real or imagined threat, the mind and body go through the fight or flight response. When someone experiences a stressful event, the area of the brain that engages the emotional processing, the amygdala, sends a distress signal to the hypothalamus. This signal elicits the endocrine system, which alerts the different systems of the body to maximize the energy a person can use to fight or flee the particularly stressful situation. This energy to fight or flee from the stressor comes from the numerous hormones that get secreted from the glands located throughout the body via the endocrine system. See Figure 1 below which shows where the endocrine glands are located.

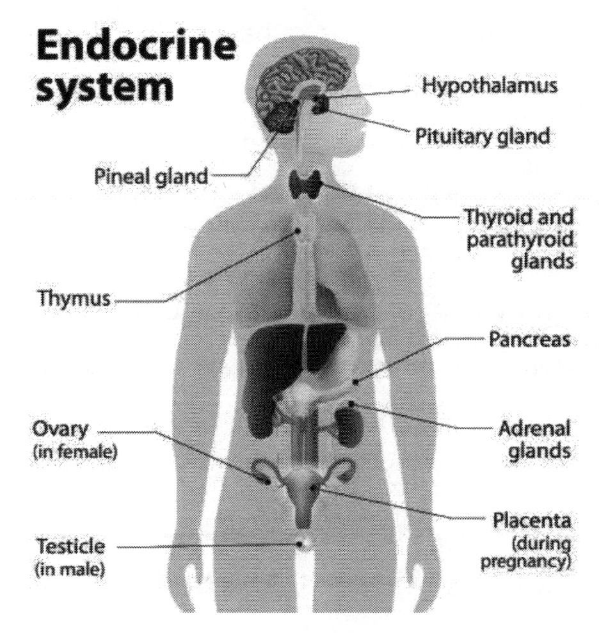

Figure 1. Location of the Endocrine Glands

The stress-related hormones that get secreted to their target organs include cortisol and adrenaline (epinephrine and norepinephrine). Cortisol and norepinephrine/epinephrine give the body the burst of energy characteristic of a fight or flight response, sometimes giving someone almost super-human strength or speed in which to deal with a stressor. These coincide with increased lung and heart activity.

Cortisol is also released slowly and continuously when we stew over problems or worry over something for extended periods of time. Although these hormones serve an important stress reactivity purpose (fight or flight for survival), the more they are secreted the more adverse response they have on a person's immune system. The stress hormones, especially cortisol and adrenaline, in time, lowers the functioning of our immune system which is in place to fight foreign substances in the body. The important point here is to limit the amount of times these hormones are secreted by being in greater control of our controllables, how we think, talk to ourselves, and how we appraise stressors.

Besides the well-researched fight or flight response, there are additional psychophysiological responses to stress, such as the shock/freeze response, the withdrawal response, and the tend-and-befriend response. In times of stress, some folks will simply freeze up, maybe due to the shock of the event and an inability to fully recognize or reason what is going on. The adage "deer in the headlights" applies here. Other people will withdraw from the stress, like a youngster who crouches into the fetal position or buries themselves under their covers when they are fearful. Tend-and-befriend is primarily a female stress response characterized by engaging in nurturing activities and communicating with others about their stressors. Males can gain the same benefits of this response, but most choose to bottle up their feelings instead and thus lose the opportunity to be more stress resilient.

The fight or flight response, along with the withdrawal and freeze responses, should only be used when absolutely needed. Too often we allow ourselves to get upset, angry, or frustrated which triggers cortisol when it really is not necessary. According to the ABC's of stress management addressed next, we have more control over our appraisals, behaviors, and responses than we believe we do.

A-B-C's of Stress Management

Referred to earlier, Hans Selye helped create a nonprofit organization, the American Institute of Stress (AIS) in 1978, which is an educational learning house for all-things stress management. Surveys from the AIS will be referenced and utilized throughout this chapter to aid in improving your awareness and knowledge of the sources of your stress, its effects on mind and body, as well as your current ability to cope with it. To aid in addressing the nine major components of stress management training and coping, an ABC list has been created and shared. The A's of SMT include awareness, assessment, and appraisals. The B's of SMT are behaviors, barriers, and balance. Whereby the C's of SMT include cognitions, control, and communication. In the next section, each will be defined and related to how they can be applied to your SMT plan.

A's of SMT

AWARENESS – To be aware of something means to know, perceive, or feel it, which may include being more aware of your surroundings, your feelings about a personal situation, or your awareness of a worry that you cannot shake. Awareness of what stresses us out as well as how we usually attempt to cope with it becomes valuable tools in the management, and even our attempts to master the stress we experience. To aid in this process is the introduction and use of assessment tools designed to educate and inform us about our predispositions (personality traits), sources of, and ways of responding/coping with stress. The activity boxes shared throughout the chapter offer more opportunities for you to increase your SMT awareness.

ASSESSMENT – Assessments come in all shapes and sizes, whether they be paper/pen surveys, on-line point and click surveys, or even self-reflection journaling or question/answer. They can all help to teach us something new or confirm our original thoughts about ourselves and how/why we think and act the way we do, especially in the face of stressors. The first assessment survey shared in this chapter comes from the AIS. It is a *360 stress assessment survey* which inquiries about your lifestyle, attitude, and diet to determine your stress load. Sample items are shared below. Your instructor may have you complete the full survey.

360 Stress Assessment Survey

1. I feel like there is not enough time to get everything done.
   a. Always or almost always
   b. Very often
   c. Often
   d. Occasionally
   e. Never or almost never

2. I experience regular muscular tension in my neck, back or shoulders (without an injury).
   a. Always or almost always
   b. Very often
   c. Often
   d. Occasionally
   e. Never or almost never

3. I have a short, shallow breathing pattern or go long periods of time without focusing on mindful breathing.
   a. Always or almost always
   b. Very often
   c. Often
   d. Occasionally
   e. Never or almost never

APPRAISAL – The "power of appraisal" cannot be emphasized enough. How one appraises or perceives a stressor can be a "game changer." The ideal is to perceive or appraise any stressor. For example, perceiving an upcoming class presentation or job interview as a challenge, rather than a threat (Figure 2). When someone perceives a stressor, like a class presentation, as a threat all sorts of physical, cognitive (thoughts and self-talk), and emotional reactions occur, namely, increased heart rate, shaky arms/fingers, negative thoughts, fearing the worst will happen. This will all lead to a poor verbal performance due to forgetting one's words and a less than ideal voice. Yet when one appraises the presentation as a challenge, an opportunity to practice speaking in front of others, which everyone will have to do at some point in any occupation they choose, you may still be nervous. However, the heart rate won't elevate too high, the appendages won't shake, you will be task focused on the presentation notes, fear will not enter in, and your voice will come out sounding smooth and confident. It's that simple – choosing to approach the situation and view it as a challenge that will be good for you rather than fear it because of the possibilities of failure.

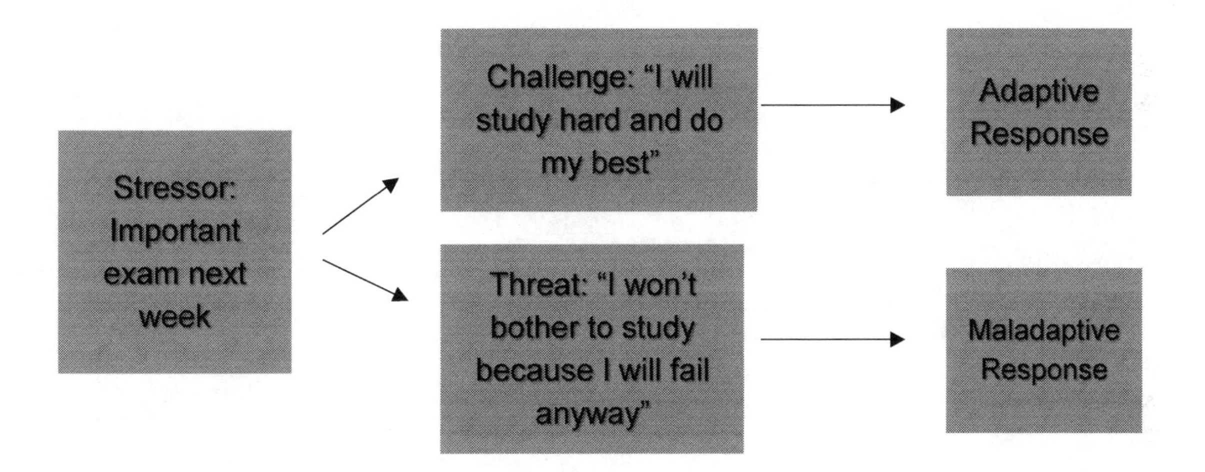

Figure 2. Appraisal of a Stressor

For practice in using the power of appraisal, see Activity #2. The term *maladaptive*, refers to thoughts and actions that are negative and self-defeating, whereby *adaptive* appraisals can motivate and inspire future productive action.

Activity #2: The Power of Appraisal

Insert how you would appraise the stressors in both maladaptive and adaptive forms. A sample is included below. Write in some recent stressors you experience and how you appraised them.

STRESSOR	MALADAPTIVE APPRAISAL	ADAPTIVE APPRAISAL
Class presentation	Oh NO! I hate doing these!	I need more experience speaking in front of people- this is a good thing
Pop Quiz		
Meeting girl/boyfriend's parents for the first time		
Job interview (For a job you really want)		

B's of SMT

BEHAVIORS – How a person behaviorally responds to stress tells a lot about the appraisal of the stressor as well as how adaptive or maladaptive the behavior is. The following information boxes include listings of maladaptive, or unhealthy, behavioral responses as well as productive responses to stress. As an In-Class Activity, highlight or circle the behaviors and responses you mostly use when in stressful situations. The more that we can use adaptive behaviors rather than maladaptive ones the better off we will be! What will you do about the maladaptive behaviors you have circled?

Maladaptive Responses

BEHAVIORS: Foot tapping, nail biting, pacing, overeating or drinking to excess; eating junk food, smoking, taking drugs or prescription meds; excessive sleeping, withdrawal; binge watching TV or streaming shows; blaming others for present situation.

MENTAL: Negative, self-defeating thoughts & self-talk; racing mind that cannot turn down or off; confusion, fatigue; depressing thoughts (hopeless, helpless); no sense of humor

EMOTIONAL: Bursts of anger & frustration; anxiety, worry, or depressed feelings; boredom; fearing failure

Adaptive Responses

BEHAVIORS: Talk with others, share your stressors; daily physical activity; consistent good rest; eat nutritious food & stay hydrated; stay on top of things by being organized; stay away from bad habits

MENTAL: Staying optimistic; embracing a hardy personality set; enjoy life, laugh often and tell those who love you that you love them! Limiting worry and regret; embrace what the future holds.

EMOTIONAL: Remain confident knowing that you can control what you can control while not trying to control the things you cannot.

In the stress management research, there is a lot of attention given to the influence that one's behavioral personality set has on one's response to stress. For example, many people have heard of the Type A personality set. This is characterized by the 3 A's: agitated, aggressive, ambitious.

Type A person gets easily agitated when things do not go smoothly, or they are put in a situation where they need to be patient. They are aggressive in how they communicate with others as they are always "confrontation ready" to prove they are right about almost any topic. Being ambitious is a good trait for the most part yet type A's take it to the extreme by doing whatever is needed to get ahead, regardless of the cost or how many people they hurt or "step on" along the way. Other behaviors portrayed by type A's can be seen in the table below (Table 1). Although some of these behaviors can help one be very productive in their occupation, once it begins to cause stress for others, these behaviors should be changed for the betterment of all involved.

The other behavioral sets include Type B, Type C, and lastly, Type R. Type A behavioral sets have been linked to increased incidence of cardiovascular disease, whereby Type C behavioral set has been indirectly linked to cancer. The term, "indirect," is used because the behaviors that characterize a Type C person can lead to a lowered immune system through psychological distress and disorders, such as anxiety and depression. According to the Psychoneuroimmunology field, a suppressed immune system has been found to lead to all sorts of cancers.

Table 1. Behavioral Sets by Personality Types

BEHAVIORAL SETS			
TYPE A	**TYPE B**	**TYPE C**	**TYPE R**
▪ 3 A's ▪ Impatient ▪ Drive ▪ Talk fast ▪ Finish other's sentences ▪ Multitasker ▪ Rigid ▪ Inflexible	▪ Balanced ▪ Assertive ▪ Confident ▪ Committed ▪ Sense of control ▪ Seeks challenges ▪ Resilient ▪ Flexible	▪ Unassertive ▪ Desire to please ▪ Believe no control ▪ Learned helplessness ▪ Learned hopelessness ▪ Anxiety & depression ▪ Fear failure	▪ Risk taking ▪ Seeks challenges ▪ Confident ▪ Sensation seeker ▪ Easily bored ▪ Embraces change ▪ Gregarious

BARRIERS – There is no limit to the barriers that people use to stay in their comfort zones. Another word for barriers could be "excuses." Think of the many barriers/excuses people come up with for not exercising on a regular basis: "no time, too expensive, I don't know what I'm doing, too far a drive, don't need it, only for muscle-heads, I'm too far gone now, it's too hard, it won't work, I have no one to exercise with, I don't too that kind of stuff." It is truly amazing how people can talk themselves in and out of just about anything. We set these barriers to keep us contained in our safe and comfortable comfort zones. Type R people are driven by the drive to experience all that life has to offer, whether that be trying new types of food, meeting new and different people, doing different activities, and simply varying up what they do from day to day. You do not have to jump out of an airplane to get all the health benefits experienced by Type R people. Not being limited by your self-prescribed barriers is a great place to start.

An exercise I have my classes do every semester is to think of their "dream" job - if you could take away all barriers that could hold you back from accomplishing it, whether it be time, money, schooling, experience, *what would you do*? The listing across the class is amazingly diverse (from being a pro athlete, to being an actress, to being a physical therapist, a pro strength coach, or running their own fitness center). When they speak of their respective dream jobs their eyes are lit up and all are smiling as they share their dream job with the class. They had this positive emotional reaction to this exercise due to the neurotransmitter, dopamine, which gets released when you have a positive appraisal for the future. Dopamine also is released when you check off tasks on your to-do list, accomplish goals, and get credit for a job well done. Being more Type R and embracing the possibilities that life provides, which entails not being limited by self-imposed barriers, will feel good (more dopamine among other neurotransmitters) because of the optimistic nature and attitudes which will drive your actions which follow. Who knows, maybe these attitudes and subsequent actions will lead you to your dream job!

BALANCE – A source of stress I often hear about in my classes is the inability to juggle all the demands college students have. From staying on top of their studies, to working part-time (some even full-time), to balancing their needs as students to the needs of their families, and maybe even their coaches and teams for the athletes. Life today is just busy. Due to technology and how often it makes our lives easier (unless it breaks down!), we can take on more and do more while always being connected to others via our smart phones, whether it be our friends, family, bosses, teachers, and anyone else who needs us. Type A's will normally focus on their own schedules and not delegate responsibilities to others, so they tend to have overly full schedules. Type C's will open their schedule up to others since they cannot say "no" and want to please everyone. Type B's are able to keep a balanced schedule, ensuring that time is scheduled for what is most important to them as well as those urgent matters that must be taken care of. There will be specific information and techniques shared in the last section of this chapter, specifically on time management. This process all starts with prioritizing what is most important to you and ensuring this gets scheduled throughout the week. Many of us do not realize that we have a lot more control over our time, and specifically our daily/weekly schedule. It is possible to balance our many life, work, school, and sport responsibilities without giving up on what makes us the happiest. Really!

C's of SMT

COGNITIONS – Cognitions refers to our thoughts and the self-talk dialogue we have with ourselves, all day, every day. Some articles have cited that we can have anywhere from 12,000 to 20,000 thoughts/self-talk statements per day. The important question is not how many you have, but the quality of them – how many are negative and self-defeating versus those that are uplifting and positive. Many people think and say to themselves the most negatives things which usually results in lowered self confidence levels, greater anxiety, and eventually, more depressive thoughts and feelings. Depression becomes a likely result of overwhelming stress when it activates a sense of helplessness, powerlessness, and hopelessness. Research has found that optimists, who have positive self-talk and belief in themselves, have better physical and psychological health than those who tend to be pessimistic with negative self-talk.

We have the control (addressed with the last "C") to alter this type of thinking from overly negative to positive and uplifting. To coincide with these negative thoughts are the irrational thoughts many folks experience, which include the following list from Dr. Albert Ellis, a cognitive psychologist who developed rational emotive behavior therapy. After reading through the list below, which of these do you think about and which rational thought should replace it?

IRRATIONAL THOUGHTS	RATIONAL THOUGHTS
"I must at all times perform great"	"Opponents can have a say about how great we play"
"Others have to approve & love me"	"Not possible- we are social creatures with all sorts of biases"
"I should get what I want"	"Not possible – as the Rolling Stones so eloquently sang, "You can't always get what you want"
"Everyone has to treat me fairly"	Fallacy of failure – how many times have your parents told you "the world is not a fair place." Sage advice
"Perfection is essential"	Striving for perfection is OK, just don't expect it; being perfect is impossible
"Worth depends on achievement"	Despite a failure you are still a good person who is loved
"Catastrophizing"	Despite a failure this is a one-time event & not permanent

CONTROL/CHOICE – Those who believe they have control over their schedules, their thoughts, and even how they feel from one moment to the next are referred to as those who have a high level of intrinsic locus of control. On the contrary, those who believe that they have little control over the events in their lives, like someone or something is "pulling the strings" score high in extrinsic locus of control. It is ideal to have an intrinsic locus of control as the greater sense of control, the greater self-determined behavior. You are in charge and you can control your reactions to stressors and adversity, physically, mentally, emotionally, and socially. Choosing to take greater control over your life, your time, your schedule, is just that – a choice. We choose to get distracted by tv, video streaming/gaming, or social media. We choose to stay on task and accomplish what needs to get done. We choose what to prioritize in our scheduling of our hours and days. When we choose to take greater control over our time and our reactions to stressors, we can achieve a balanced approach to our every day. For practice identifying what you have control over (controllables) and what you do not (uncontrollable), see the Activity #3 below.

Activity #3: Controllables vs. Uncontrollables

Insert what you believe you have control over and what you do not. Think about the many situations you find yourself in at home with your family or roommates, in classes, at practice with your sport team, and even hanging out with your friends. A sample is included.

What I have control over = CONTROLLABLES	What I do not have control over = UNCONTROLLABLES
How I respond to bad calls from referees	Referees' bad calls
(1)	
(2)	
(3)	
(4)	
(5)	

COMMUNICATION – We have already tackled the importance of communicating compassionately with ourselves via our internal thoughts and self-talk to keep us more confident, motivated, and more stress resilient. This is referred to as intrapersonal communication. Ensuring that our communication with others is as productive as possible (called interpersonal communication), via the effective sending and receiving of information, along with ensuring that our nonverbal communication aligns with the spoken word, will greatly lessen the stress experienced by both parties.

Think for a moment how much stress is created during some recent communication breakdowns you have experienced (people not listening, people not connecting or communicating well enough). The stress can be experienced by all involved. Usually during communication breakdowns feelings can be hurt and the tension and stress may continue to elevate into arguments and confrontations, which unfortunately could lead to long-term feuds. This also includes being a good listener, which means that you are not trying to rush the person to the finish (like a type A would do) but rather giving the person your total attention, including facing them, making eye contact, and even paraphrasing what they have told you: "So what you think is the best course of action is for us to ...." Techniques such as these will ensure that the information sent and received occurs, thus eliminating miscommunication which can cause a lot of stress and discontent.

Sources of Stress and Coping Methods

Sources of Stress

If you completed the full 360 Stress Assessment Survey you will have a sense of what stresses you out. For even more specific information about these and more sources of your stress, complete Activity #4. The activity includes the College Re-adjustment Rating Scale, which is from Rutgers University who adapted the Holmes and Rahe's Life Events Scale. According to Stress and the College Student newsletter published by the National Health Ministries, it has been modified for college-age adults and should be considered as a rough indication of stress levels that can have possible health consequences.

Activity #4: College Re-adjustment Rating Scale

Each event in the table below, such as one's first term in college, is assigned a point value that represents the amount of readjustment a person must make.

To determine your stress score, circle the points corresponding to the events you experienced in the past 6 months or are likely to experience in the next 3 months. Then add up the circled numbers and record your answer in the total column.

EVENT	POINTS
Death of significant other	100
Female unwed pregnancy	92
Death of a parent	80
Male partner in unwed pregnancy	77
Divorced parents	73
Death of a family member	70
Death of a close friend	65
Death of beloved pet	63
Legal issues	61
Major personal injury or illness	60
Marriage	55
Fired from a job	50
Loss of financial support from college	48
Failing grade in important or required class	47
Daily hassles (commute traffic, same stressors daily)	45
Serious argument with significant other	40

-continue to next page

EVENT	POINTS
Academic probation	39
Change in major	37
New love interest	36
Increased workload from college	31
Outstanding personal achievement	29
First term in college	28
Serious conflict with instructor	27
Lower than expected grades	25
Change in college (transfer)	24
Change in social activities	22
Change in sleeping habits	21
Change in eating habits	19
Minor violations of the law (i.e. traffic ticket)	15
TOTAL:	

1. Persons with scores of 300 and higher have a high health risk and might consider seeking professional assistance to manage stress.
2. Persons scoring between 150 and 300 have about a 50 - 50 chance of serious health change within two years and may want to do frequent stress self-checks to be certain they are coping as well as they think they are.
3. People scoring 150 and below have a 1 in 3 chance of a serious health change but should still consider stress reduction activities.

Source: http://healthnet.rutgers.edu/stress/stressed_out.asp
Stress and The College Student - National Health Ministries - PC (USA).

Ways of Responding to Stress

Now that you are more *aware* of your sources of stress, and hopefully from this point forward will make a more conscious effort to control those you can control, the next focus point is on how best to respond to stress. Let's turn to another activity:

Activity #5: How Do You Respond to Stress?

(From NAS Database, 'Stress Management for the Health of It')

The following is a list of symptoms that are the most typical reactions to stress. Check all that apply to you when you are stressed, then go through and circle the ones that occur the most frequently. After completing, ask yourself: Do any patterns emerge? Which of these reactions concern you? Which coping method can be effective with each of the stress reactions that concern you? Read through the Coping section next to best answer this last question.

PHYSICAL:

__ headaches
__ fatigue
__ insomnia
__ weight change
__ colds
__ digestive upsets
__ accident-prone
__ teeth grinding
__ restlessness
__ increased alcohol, drug, tobacco use
__ neck and shoulders tighten up/ache
__ pounding heart

MENTAL:

__ forgetfulness
__ dull senses
__ poor concentration
__ low productivity
__ negative attitude
__ confusion
__ lethargy
__ no new ideas
__ boredom

EMOTIONAL:

__ anxiety
__ the "blues"
__ moods swings
__ bad temper
__ crying spells
__ irritability
__ depression
__ nervous laugh
__ worrying
__ easily discouraged

SOCIAL:

__ isolation
__ resentment
__ loneliness
__ lashing out
__ lowered sex drive
__ nagging
__ fewer contacts with friends
__using / manipulating people
__ clamming up

Ways of Coping

According to psychologist Richard Lazarus, coping is a dynamic process consisting of cognitions and behaviors used to manage external or internal demands or stressors. There are numerous types of coping, along with specific strategies, see below:

- ✓ **PROBLEM FOCUSED COPING** – use of activities specific to getting tasks done so to remove or reduce the stressor, such as dividing the task up into little segments, rewarding oneself upon completion, and managing the study environment and time management practices. This works best as it attempts to eliminate the cause of the stressor, whereby emotion focused may help make one feel better about the stressor but in most cases the stressor has not been removed.

- ✓ **EMOTION FOCUSED COPING** – use of activities to feel better about the task. These can include distraction (keeping yourself busy or any number of distractions, like social media), game playing, eating comfort food and drinking, or more positive activities such as meditation or journaling. Some will use emotion focused coping to prepare themselves productively for a task, such as setting up the studying environment (quite space, room to spread their papers out, and comfortable seating) so they feel comfortable and ready to work. In most cases, however, emotional focused is used as a distraction or procrastination.

- ✓ **APPRAISAL FOCUSED COPING** – appraising the stressor as a challenge rather than a threat; this also encompasses keeping things in perspective and looking to the idealistic future. Ideal strategies to maximize this type of coping is reflection, journaling, and using one's social support to confide in and share thoughts and feelings.

- ✓ **AVOIDANCE FOCUSED COPING** – Those who, and there are so many out there, who procrastinate and put off doing tasks practice this type of coping. Usually we procrastinate tasks that makes us feel bad about ourselves due to the challenge of the task and our lack of self-belief that we can accomplish it at a quality-enough level. We also avoid tasks simply because we are bored and want to do other things. You are practicing avoidance focused coping when coming up with excuses for not exercising, or showing up to class, or completing an assignment.

- ✓ **FAILURE TO COPE** – Those who simply choose to not deal or cope. These people will stay in bed or call in sick to steer clear of the environment or situation, like attending classes.

The next section will detail additional stress management techniques, primarily physical and cognitive-relaxation techniques. The last strategy, behavioral, will be addressed in the last section, time management.

Stress Management Intervention Strategies

Physical Interventions

PHYSICAL ACTIVITY. One of the most salient stress management strategies is that of physical activity. As referenced earlier, in times of stress, numerous fight or flight hormones are secreted into the blood stream which is not a good thing for the body or the immune system under repeated bouts. But when one exercises as a stress management technique, these stress hormones are "taken on a walk, run, lift" or any other forms of activity and used in a productive manner. These hormones are used instead as a form of energy. Physical activity also induces the "feel good" neurotransmitters like *serotonin*, which impacts mood state (antidepressant effect actually), improved sleep, memory, appetite and digestion, and *endorphins* that dull our perceptions of pain and leads to feeling of positivity and exhilaration (like type R's experience). It has been indicated that singing and dancing releases the neurotransmitter, oxytocin, which evokes feelings of pride, gratitude, appreciation, belonging, and satisfaction.

Physical fitness and participation sports are positively associated with mental health, well-being, and stress resiliency, including the reduction of anxiety, depression, fears of failure, muscle tension, resting heart rate, and stress hormones such as cortisol. There are many additional benefits of physical activity, all of which positively impact the 8 wellness dimensions = emotional, spiritual, intellectual, physical, environmental, financial, occupational, and social wellness.

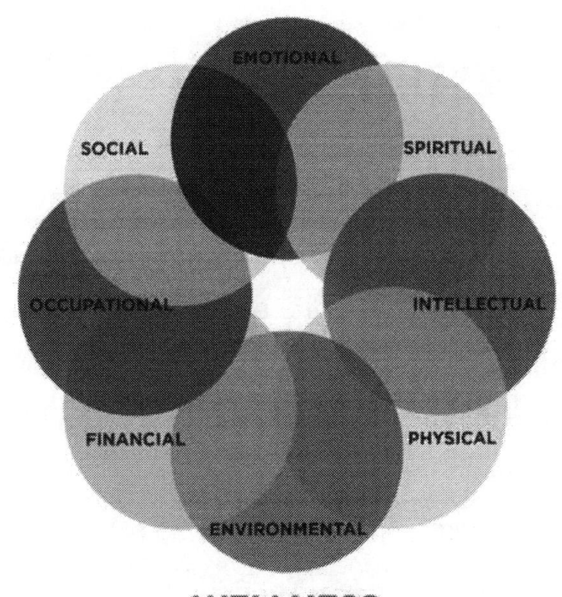

NUTRITION/HYDRATION. As stated previously, one of the maladaptive reactions to stress is to overeat and/or consume comfort foods, usually those loaded with carbohydrates, fats, and sugars, and/or to drink caffeinated and sugary beverages, including juices, sodas, coffee, alcohol, energy drinks, and sports drinks. Foods and substances like these add lots of calories to our daily intake, can dehydrate you, and could lead to even more medical issues. For example, recent studies have shown that energy drinks can lead to what the World Health Agency stated, "may pose danger to public health," and the Academy of Pediatrics reported that "children should not consume them." Moreover, when energy drinks are mixed with alcohol, studies have shown that those who do this are more inclined to engage in risk-taking behaviors and linked to numerous deleterious health effects, like high blood pressure and heart function.

Additional ways that stress and nutrition relate is that some foods and substances can mimic the stress response. These are referred to as pseudo stressors, which elicit similar fight or flight stress hormones being secreted, such as caffeine, nicotine from cigarettes, salt, sugars, and fats. Moreover, stress hormones, such as cortisol, require vitamins (primarily the B-complex and vitamin C) to do what they do in the body which gets depleted in longer durations of the stress response. Deficiencies in these vitamins can lead to depression, anxiety, insomnia, and muscular weakness.

Relaxation Interventions

RELAXATION BREATHING. Most us only breath with our thoracic breath where we expand the upper and middle costals of the chest, usually low air volume per breath. The ideal is to use our diaphragm in the abdomen, where we expand the belly on the inhale through the nose for a count of five, then exhale out the mouth to a count of five. This way we are getting a full breath and maximizing the lung capacity.

According to Healthy Living, "Breaths taken while stomach breathing are slow and deep, taking longer to inhale and exhale, and deliver a significantly larger amount of oxygen to the bloodstream. The larger amount of air intake also allows you to exhale a larger amount of carbon dioxide, eliminating it from your body at a faster rate." Try practicing relaxation breathing when you feel stressed.

PROGRESSIVE RELAXATION. This relaxation technique is a mind-body process of moving from the stress response to the relaxation response via self-induced tension then relaxation cycles. The many documented benefits of progressive relaxation include slowing the heart rate (less work for heart), reduced blood pressure, slow rate of breathing, lessen muscle tension, fewer illness symptoms, more energy, improved concentration, better able to handle adversity, and less stress prone.

Important practice considerations for progressive relaxation include: finding a quiet place with no interruptions, practice for 10-20 minutes per day, do not try too hard, just let it happen, and do not hurry to the end. Many progressive relaxation routines begin with tightening muscle groups (in the feet, for example), then after holding onto the tension, release it to induce relaxation. Then tense muscles in the lower leg and after holding onto the tension, release that. Then move on up the body tensing, holding, and relaxing, all the way up the body to the forehead. This toe-to-head cycle is an excellent pre-nap or pre-bedtime routine to induce sleep in a quick and efficient manner. After much practice, the idea is to develop good enough awareness whereby after tensing one muscle group then relaxing it, the relaxation can be felt across the body while also quieting the mind.

AUTOGENIC TRAINING. This relaxation exercise was first developed by a German psychiatrist, Dr. Johannes Shultz. It is designed to induce the relaxation response by imagining and feeling the sensations of heaviness and warmth in our musculature. According to WebMD.com, "Autogenic training consists of six standard exercises that make the body feel warm, heavy, and relaxed. For each exercise, you get into a simple posture (sitting in a comfortable chair or reclining), concentrate without any goal, and then use visual imagination and verbal cues to relax your body in some specific way." Similar to progressive relaxation, this sequence is usually done from one part of the body to the next, and it is important also to find a quiet place where you will not be interrupted. It is recommended to avoid eating and drinking prior to practicing any of these relaxation techniques as it will interfere with the relaxation process. It is ideal to keep a certain amount of awareness about you, so you do not fall asleep during the practice, unless it is done prior to bedtime and this is one of the goals you have set for this program. This technique does take more focus and practice than others do to get the full benefits, but there are similar benefits to doing this as have been found for yoga and progressive relaxation.

MEDITATION. Meditation is a mental state characterized by stillness, concentration, and being in the moment. It is one of many methods of mindfulness-based stress management strategies that has been found effective in helping people handle heart disease, cancer, chronic pain, insomnia, anxiety, depression, and others. Kottler and

Chen (2011) indicated being mindful "means sensitizing yourself to what is going on NOW" and that meditation is a way of seeing, feeling, knowing and a way of loving, both yourself and others (p. 216). There are many different types of meditation, including transcendental meditation, visual meditation, and walking meditation, yet there are thousands of different meditation forms throughout the world. Some of the common elements to effective meditative practice includes a quite environment, a comfortable position or posture, an object to focus upon, like a word or mantra, and a poised awareness (if your attention wanders, just bring it back to the present).

YOGA. Yoga is an ancient form of exercise which originated in India which consists of holding certain postures combined with breathing and relaxation exercises. Yoga can help accomplish many things, including: developing mind-body connection, positive thoughts and self- acceptance, helps heal other traumas, heightens creativity and concentration, and provides tools for everyday life. Hatha Yoga is said to be the most popular type of yoga.

There are six common principles to yoga practice:

1) Proper relaxation = relaxed body, focused mind, spiritual relaxation
2) Proper exercise = asanas and postures
3) Proper breathing = inhale, retention, exhalation
4) Proper diet
5) Positive thinking & meditation = mantras, chants
6) Good deeds (altruism)

There are many videos on-line that can take you through a yoga session or find a nearby yoga studio and take a class that can count towards your activity assignment as part of this class!

Behavioral Interventions

TIME FLIES – HOW TO MANAGE YOUR TIME AND SCHEDULE. According to Kottler and Chen (2011), authors of *Stress Management and Prevention,* "Time management is actually a form of life management. Controlling your life means controlling your time, and controlling your time means controlling the events in your life" (p. 183). It is truly amazing how important our time has become in this very hectic world we live in. Being able to manage our time via what we prioritize and how we schedule our responsibilities is almost an art form these days. This section challenges you to become more aware of *how* we spend our time currently and *what* changes must be made to not only be efficient and productive with our time but to also live a more balanced life.

To gain this awareness, Elkin (1999) suggested answering the open-ended questions below.

- ✓ Do you have enough time to do the things that are most important to you?
- ✓ Do you feel bored or restless much of the time?
- ✓ Are you rushing to complete tasks and often get things done at the last minute?
- ✓ Do you have enough time to do the things you enjoy the most?
- ✓ Do you not plan and prioritize the most urgent things you need to accomplish?
- ✓ Do you say "no" to people who make demands of your time that is beyond what you can usually handle?

According to Elkin (1999), if you answered "no" to more than a couple of these questions is an indicator that you have some time management issues.

Another awareness exercise comes from a volleyball coach from USC who taught me this *dot exercise* (Activity #6). The idea is to cross out a dot for every hour spent during your day attending classes, working out, studying, eating, hanging out, playing games, sport training, working, and anything else you spend your time doing throughout a 24-hour period. Do Activity #6 below for several days (make copies of the dot chart below so you can complete it for several days). It will become quite apparent how little time you have left over in your day, especially if you have not prioritized the most important things into your daily schedules.

Activity #6: The DOT Exercise

There are 24 dots below. Cross out a dot for ***every hour*** spent during your day attending classes, working out, studying, eating, hanging out, playing games, sport training, working, and anything else you spend your time doing throughout a 24-hour period. Notice how many dots you have left at the end of the day. Complete this for several days.

Day 1

○ ○ ○ ○ ○ ○ ○ ○ ○ ○ ○ ○

○ ○ ○ ○ ○ ○ ○ ○ ○ ○ ○ ○

Day 2

○ ○ ○ ○ ○ ○ ○ ○ ○ ○ ○ ○

○ ○ ○ ○ ○ ○ ○ ○ ○ ○ ○ ○

Day 3

○ ○ ○ ○ ○ ○ ○ ○ ○ ○ ○ ○

○ ○ ○ ○ ○ ○ ○ ○ ○ ○ ○ ○

See the "Tips" box below for additional strategies to best manage your time and schedule by fighting your time zapper and procrastination habits. Keep in mind the 80-20 rule: 80% of what you do may contribute only 20% of what you actually achieve. To reframe it, 20% of tasks we do give 80% of rewards-satisfaction, so give special attention to those most important goals and projects that can really make a huge difference in your schooling and future career and life.

TIME ZAPPER AND OVERCOMING PROCRASTINATION TIPS:

- Most of the time we procrastinate those things that are not important to us. Change your outlook on those activities and reward yourself if needed to accomplish it.
- Reminding yourself that the more you put things off the more stress you will experience and the less likely you will ever want to do it. Do it now and reward yourself for doing it.
- Divide the project or task into smaller, more manageable parts, and begin this work earlier- "turn elephants into hors d'oeuvres"
- Avoid cramming. Taking breaks while working and studying will only improve the process and product
- Manage time zappers by using them as rewards (social media, tv, games)
- Work hardest during your "best times" of the day
- Choose to refuse= say NO when you do not have time to take on anything else
- Do the most difficult or unpleasant tasks first

Chapter Summary

✓ Hans Selye, a pioneer in the study of stress, defined stress as the "nonspecific response of the body to any demand made upon it."

✓ Stress can sometimes be confused with anxiety and arousal. When a stressor is perceived as a threat to one's self esteem or in the rare occurrence, a physical threat, it produces extreme psychological and emotional reactions which could include anxiety, fear, frustration, anger, depression, or other negative emotional and mood states.

- ✓ In times of adversity, especially when one appraises a stressor as a real or imagined threat, the mind and body go through the fight or flight response. The energy to fight or flee from the stressor comes from the numerous hormones that get secreted from the glands located throughout the body via the endocrine system.
- ✓ To aid in addressing the nine major components of stress management training and coping, an ABC list has been created and shared. The A's of SMT include awareness, assessment, and appraisals. The B's of SMT are behaviors, barriers, and balance, whereby the C's of SMT include cognitions, control, and communication. In the next section, each will be defined and related to how each can be applied to your SMT plan.
- ✓ There is a lot of attention given to the influence that one's behavioral personality set has on one's response to stress. For example, many people have heard of the Type A personality set. This is characterized by the 3 A's: agitated, aggressive, ambitious. The other behavioral sets include Type B, Type C, and Type R.
- ✓ According to psychologist Richard Lazarus, coping is a dynamic process consisting of cognitions and behaviors used to manage external or internal demands or stressors. The different types of coping include: problem focused, emotion focused, appraisal focused, avoidance focused, and failure to cope.
- ✓ There are numerous stress management intervention techniques, including physical interventions, relaxation techniques, and behavioral strategies which include time management and procrastination-busting practices.

Chapter Review Questions

1) Define stress.
2) Describe some examples of recent distress and eustress stressors you have experienced.
3) Identify the different stress responses.
4) Explain the fight or flight response and the significant hormones that get secreted.
5) Identify the A–B–C's of stress management addressed in this chapter.
6) List some of the more common irrational thoughts people say/think to themselves. Next to these, write an alternative rational thought to use instead.
7) Describe your most common ways of responding to the stress you experience.
8) Detail the different stress management techniques and which ones you will begin to incorporate into your stress management practices.

Website Resources and Professional Organizations

- ✓ American Heart Association (AHA) -
  - **www.heart.org/HEARTORG/HealthyLiving/StressManagement/**
- ✓ American Institute of Stress (AIS)
  - **www.stress.org**
- ✓ American Psychological Association (APA)
  - **www.apa.org/topics/stress/**
- ✓ Global Organization for Stress (GOStress)
  - **www.gostress.com**
- ✓ International Stress Management Association (ISMA)
  - **http://isma.org.uk**
- ✓ National Cancer Institute
  - **www.cancer.gov**

References

Elkin, A. (1999). *Stress Management for Dummies*. New York: Wiley.

Greenberg, J. (2013). *Comprehensive Stress Management*, 13th ed. New York: McGraw Hill.

Kottler, J. A. & Chen, D. (2011). *Stress Management and Prevention*, 2nd ed. New York: Routledge.

Lazarus, R. S. & Folkman, S. (1984). *Stress, Appraisal, and Coping.* New York: Springer.

Chapter 8

Financial Wellness

By Jan Galen Bishop, EdD and Richard Bishop, MSA

Chapter Objectives

After reading this chapter, students should be able to:

- ✓ Manage financial resources effectively with a goal of creating lifetime financial security;
- ✓ Explain the 5 components of financial literacy;
- ✓ Create and follow a weekly/monthly budget;
- ✓ Build good credit and know how to monitor it;
- ✓ Enter loans with consumer knowledge and a repayment plan;
- ✓ Protect against financial fraud; and
- ✓ Know where to find food and financial assistance on campus.

Financial Wellness

"A penny saved is a penny earned" - Benjamin Franklin

Financial well-being is having monetary security and freedom for both the present and the future. Owning the skills and habits to control your day-to-day and month-to-month finances will allow you to handle short-term expenses and provide the means to finance your long-term goals. Financial wellness also means being protected from unexpected financial surprises so that you stay on track and experience less stress when/if difficulties arise.

This chapter will explain the steps to financial literacy, how to develop and monitor a budget, what to consider when taking on loans, what you need to know about using credit, and developing a good credit history and score, and how to manage costs and contracts when setting up your own apartment.

Financial Literacy

Financial literacy refers to the set of skills and knowledge that allows an individual to make informed and effective decisions with all their financial resources (National Financial Educators Council, 2013).

There are 3 steps to becoming financially literate. You must:

1) **BE COMMITTED.** Acknowledge that your actions and attitude towards money, will drive your habits in spending and saving and investing. You need to take responsibility for your finances.

2) **ASSESS YOUR SITUATION.** Examine your core earnings, savings, spending, and borrowing, as well as how you are protecting yourself from financial troubles. You will need to document your financial practices and consider ways

to improve your earnings, savings and investments. You will also need to develop a plan for protecting yourself (and family) with insurance and ultimately for retirement.

3) **BECOME ORGANIZED.** Develop a good budget that you can sustain and is simple enough that you will follow it. Your budget should allow for items that you need and some you don't need but want, and still allow for your security.

Financial literacy has 5 basic competencies, all of which need to be understood and applied when managing your money. They are:

✓ **EARNING.** This refers to the money you make at work. Your paycheck will list gross and net earnings and it is important to understand the difference. The gross income is the total amount you earn before any deductions. So if you work 10 hours at $10/hour, your gross income would be $100. However, the average employee will pay between 28%-30% of their gross income in taxes and other deductions. What is left is the net income which in this example would be about $70. Budgeting must be based on the net income. As you explore college majors and career choices, it is important to consider and understand future earning potentials, but salary potential should not be the only criteria.

✓ **SAVINGS AND INVESTING.** This pertains to the understanding of financial institutions and services. You should have a checking and savings account to manage your finances. Start saving early by putting money into savings and investments. It is important to learn how to invest and grow your money over time.

✓ **SPENDING**. One of the most important skills to learn is spending - because it is personal to you. You need to know the difference between needs and wants and use this information as the basis of spending. Budgeting will be one of the most important tools you can develop to control spending and allow for saving and investing in your future.

- ✓ **BORROWING.** Most students will borrow student loans to finance their college education. Having a good repayment plan will be an advantage to you in the future. Borrowing for education is an investment in your future. Taking a mortgage to buy a home or other borrowing such as a business loan to create a self-employment opportunity are also examples of how borrowing can be turned into an asset and grow wealth.

- ✓ **PROTECTING.** You will want to be financially protected in multiple ways. Protecting yourself and your family through risk management involves things like health and property insurance and protection from identify theft, fraud, and scams.

Earning

Decisions you make now will impact your earning power in both the short- and long-term. Most immediate for many students is to earn enough money to pay for tuition and fees, room and board, and books. This may require working year-round if summer earnings and family support are not enough. (If you are fortunate enough to not have to fund your own education, it is still important to learn how to handle earnings and budgeting to attain future goals.)

Student employment is very convenient as it involves jobs right on campus, they require no transportation, and work well with class schedules. The two typical types of student employment are Federal Work Study and Student Labor. Federal Work Study requires you to apply for financial aid, be determined eligible, and then awarded work study by the Financial Aid Office. Student Labor positions do not require students to be eligible for financial aid. There are Student Labor positions available in many departments on campus. The listings for both Federal Work Study and Student Labor are on the College Central Network at **www.collegecentral.com/ccsu/**.

The Career Success Center at CCSU can assist you in finding work on campus, discipline-related internships, and career employment after graduation. The resources and services provided through this office include: 1-on-1 Career Coaching, Resume/Cover Letter Critiques, Internships, Co-ops, Job Search Strategies, Interview Preparation and Practice, Career Development Workshops, Networking with Employers, and Career Fairs. Financial security can be obtained by planning for a career while still taking classes. An additional benefit is that the CCSU Career Success Center is also available to alumni.

Savings and Earnings: Budgeting

Why Do You Need a Budget?

Have you ever found yourself looking at your bank account balance wondering where your money went? The most common cause of financial problems is spending more than what you are earning. How can you avoid being in this situation? Creating a flexible, sensible budget is the best way to ensure that you are in control of your money. A budget is simply a plan for how you will spend your money. It can help you restrict your spending, but it can also help you ensure that there is enough money to do the things that you want to do. Think of it as a roadmap to help you carry out your financial objectives.

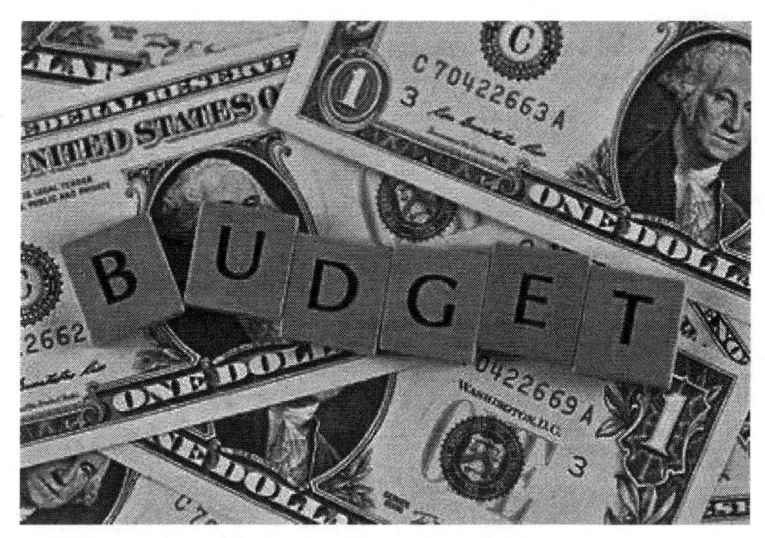

The Principles of Budgeting

The purpose of budgeting is to manage your earnings and spending. A balanced budget spends the same amount as earned. This does not mean you should spend everything you earn in order to balance your budget. Putting money in savings is considered "spending," so good budgeting is to put some money in savings, spend on essentials, and only then on non-essentials with the money you have left. If your budget is out of balance, you have 2 choices - either increase your earnings or decrease spending. The obvious way to increase earnings is to work more hours or obtain a job that pays better. Other possibilities are to turn a hobby into a money generating activity, get seasonal work, or invest in stocks and bonds to earn dividends. You can also choose to rent out a room if living in a house or rent storage or garage space. With enough capital, you can invest in real estate to get rental income. Some individuals do well buying items cheap and reselling them on sites like eBay for a profit. The other way to balance a budget and be free of debt is to decrease spending. To do this, you first need to find out where you are spending your money and determine if you are prioritizing your spending correctly (needs vs. wants).

Activity #1: Needs versus Wants

- ✓ "**NEEDS**" are items/products, or services you must have in order to be healthy and safe.
- ✓ "**WANTS**" are things you enjoy but don't have to have.

Write down where you spend money under each category.

i.e. Electric bill (need), Movie Ticket (want)

NEEDS	WANTS

To set up a budget, you usually want to work with monthly earnings and spending as some bills such as rent and car payments only occur once a month. Use your best guess of what you spend in a month. Write this down. Here are some categories you might use: books, personal expenses, rent, food, telephone and entertainment. Then, track your expenses for a month - you can use a piece of paper, a computer spreadsheet, or budgeting app. At the end of the month compare your estimate to your actual spending. You may be surprised to see where your guesses were higher or lower than your actual spending.

Once you have tracked your expenses for a month, total up all of your expenses and subtract them from your income. If you are spending more than you are earning, you will need to make changes. Look at your spending pattern and sort your "needs" and your "wants". Be honest about what a necessity is and isn't. (Enjoying a fancy coffee every day is nice, but you could save yourself $80-120 a month by only having it once a week.) Cut back on the "wants" either gradually or cold turkey depending on your commitment to being debt free. Also look at your needs to see if there is a way to reduce spending there (i.e. taking in a roommate, planning errands better to cut back on gas, etc.) List any changes you plan on making in your budget. Be sure that you are balancing your spending against your take-home (net) pay. Review your budget monthly to see if there are any changes you may need or want to make. Careful budgeting will allow you to include more "wants" over time, but always try to keep some money tucked away for a rainy day.

Activity #2: Track your Weekly Spending

Use the Tracking Sheet on the next page to track your spending for one week.

Ask yourself:

- ✓ What do you spend most of your money on?
- ✓ Are you spending more than you have?
- ✓ How can you cut back on any excessive spending?
- ✓ How can you save?

MONDAY		TUESDAY		WEDNESDAY		THURSDAY		FRIDAY		SATURDAY		SUNDAY	
ITEM	COST	ITEM	COST	ITEM	COST	ITEM	COST	ITEM	COST	ITEM	COST	ITEM	COST

Saving and Investing

The way to gain financial security is by saving and investing. As a college student, these are topics that are not likely on your radar at this time. But saving is a key principle, so if you make saving a habit now, even if it's a small amount, you are building a foundation for financial success.

Moving Forward with a Flexible Budget

For your budget to be useful, and not just a piece of scrap paper, you need to follow it. Recording your purchases at the end of the day should only take a few minutes. (If you use a budgeting app that links to your checking and credit card accounts and automatically imports and categorizes your purchases, the process is even easier.) If you are finding it hard to stick to your budget on a regular basis, some of your figures may have been unrealistic. Go back over your budget and make adjustments. Perhaps you realize you need to allocate more money towards books and school supplies, and that you are able to spend less money on clothing. The best budget is one that can grow and change to meet your needs.

Budgeting Tips

PUT YOURSELF FIRST! You've probably heard this before. This means that for every paycheck you receive, you commit to putting an amount (even a small amount) aside in a savings account. The most effective way of doing this is by having your paycheck directly deposited into an account and then set up an automatic transfer, with your financial institution, into a separate savings account.

KEEP TRACK OF YOUR SAVING. People who track their savings tend to save more because they feel good watching it grow. With online and mobile banking, as well as a variety of apps, it is easy to know exactly how much money you have.

SET GOALS. Setting financial goals is a key component of staying on the path to getting what you want. As a student, you may have very limited financial goals, but this is the perfect opportunity to practice the process.

Creating a Budget for Living on Your Own

Either during college or after graduating from college, a common goal is to live on your own (choosing an apartment). The challenges of living on your own are often not the same as the expectation. This section is to provide a little reality check for you as you investigate the costs of moving, renting an apartment, appliances, obtaining furniture.

In preparation, remember the budgeting process. Remember budgeting strategies for both flexible expenses (variable costs that change depending on level of consumption), such as entertainment, restaurants, and vacations, and fixed expenses (those that need to be paid every month), such as rent and apartment insurance.

As you start the apartment selection process, many items need to be considered. Costs will vary based on where you live, for rent and transportation to and from your home, the type of lease (month to month are more expensive than yearly contracts), and whether you choose to live alone or share the apartment with another person. Read the lease carefully and be sure you understand the rights and legal responsibilities of a tenant and a landlord. Parking and utilities may cost extra. Set up a budget that includes rent, moving expenses, and the expenses associated with setting up a household.

Typical costs associated with living on your own are included in the following table:

<table>
<tr><td><u>TYPICAL FIXED MONTHLY EXPENSES</u>
✓ Rent
✓ Car payment
✓ Car insurance</td><td><u>MOVING COSTS</u>
✓ Renting a truck or hiring movers
✓ Packing supplies</td></tr>
<tr><td><u>TYPICAL FLEXIBLE MONTHLY EXPENSES</u>
✓ Food
✓ Utilities
✓ Transportation (gas, bus, Uber, etc.)
✓ Clothing
✓ Entertainment
✓ Personal items</td><td rowspan="2"><u>APARTMENT FURNISHING COSTS</u>
✓ Furniture
✓ Kitchen
✓ Bedroom(s)
✓ Living Room
✓ Dining Room
✓ Rugs
✓ Linens (bed and bath)
✓ Electronics/Appliances
✓ Dishes/Pans/Utensils
✓ Other</td></tr>
<tr><td>RENTAL COSTS
✓ Rent for first/last month
✓ Cleaning/Security deposit
✓ Utilities deposit</td></tr>
</table>

There are ways to cut costs, such as purchasing used furnishings and equipment from secondhand stores, online, and in local newspapers. Relatives may also be able to give you used furniture. It is also cheaper to move yourself than hiring someone. Another option is to share an apartment with one or several people. If you are considering sharing an apartment or home, it is a good idea to make certain decisions up front so that all involved feel that it is fair.

- ✓ Lifestyle compatibility
- ✓ How to split expenses
- ✓ How to divide chores
- ✓ House rules
- ✓ Legal obligations if someone moves out

Borrowing

There are three common ways in which students borrow money. One is the use of credit cards which when used well can build a good credit record but if used poorly can result in overpaying through high interest rates. The second is taking out student loans to pay for college expenses. The third is taking out loans for things such the purchase of a car. The first two are discussed in this chapter. The third requires careful reading of the contract as is beyond the scope of this chapter.

Credit: Financial Success

In today's economy credit is one of the most important factors, the better your credit score the better position you will be in. A good credit score is important for buying a car with favorable terms, obtaining your own cell phone account, renting an apartment or buying a home.

What is a Credit Report vs. Credit Score?

A credit report is a very detailed and nearly complete history of all your credit. It will show your personal information, employment history, and list of open and closed credit accounts. You should review your credit report at least once per year for accuracy and check for fraud. You can obtain a free copy of your credit report up to three times per year, one from each of the major credit reporting agencies. By checking your credit report, you will be able to identify if someone has opened a credit card or obtained credit using your information.

Your credit score (also called your FICO score) is a snapshot of your credit risk at a specific point in time. It is based on your current credit report and is designed to allow lenders to quickly assess your credit worthiness. FICO scores range from 300-850. The higher the score, the lower the chance of a default (failure to fulfill your financial obligation). Building a solid credit history will make you eligible for lower interest rates on various credit products such as private school loans, credit cards, auto loans, and insurance. You can check your credit (FICO) score yourself through your bank or online (See Activity #3)

Activity #3: Check Your FICO Score

Check your credit score online at:

www.annualcreditreport.com

You can obtain a free copy of your credit report up to three times per year, one from each of the major credit reporting agencies

What Makes Up Your Credit Score?

Payment history makes up the largest component, 35%, of your credit score. The best way for you to improve your credit score is by making consistent on-time payments. If you are more than 30 days late even once, that record will remain on your credit report for 7 years and could result in a drop of 90+ points in your credit score.

The amount of debt you have relative to how much credit you have makes up 30% of your score. Keep the amounts owed / total credit limit below 30%. For example, if you have a credit card with a $2,000 credit limit, you should only charge $600.

How long you have had a credit history makes up 15% of the score. Lenders like to see that you have long time history with other lenders. One of the easiest things you can do to build your credit history is to open a credit card with no annual fee, charge a few dollars, then pay it off every month. If you manage your credit responsibly, you can earn a high credit score with a short credit history.

Establishing new credit makes up 10% of your score. When you apply for a new credit card, at a store or bank (consumer loan etc.), your credit score drops by 2-5 points. This is something to remember the next time you are at a store and they ask you if you want to save 10% by applying for their store credit card. This information remains on your credit report for 2 years. Having 1-2 credit cards you use regularly is generally healthier than having a large number of store specific cards. If you shop a lot at one store and the rewards program significantly benefits you, then that may be worthwhile.

The mix in the type of credit you have makes up 10% of the score. Creditors like to see a variety of credit accounts because it tells them that you are a responsible borrower. A person who is making monthly payments on a credit card, an auto loan, and a student loan is deemed to be less risky which is why this component is included in your score.

Are You Ready for a Credit Card?

To determine if you're ready for a credit card, ask yourself the following questions:

- ✓ Do you impulse buy often?
- ✓ Do you spend more per week than you earn?

If you answer yes to either of these questions, then getting a credit card might not be a good idea for you at this time. You should wait until you get your spending under control. It is best to pay off your credit card in full every month. If you can do that, you will not have to pay any interest, and can build your credit history.

Types of Money Cards

CREDIT CARD — A credit card lets you buy things and pay for them over time. Buying with credit is a loan; you must pay the money back. Some credit card issuers charge an annual fee, others do not. Some credit card issuers also provide "courtesy" checks to you. You can use these checks in place of your card, but they're not a gift, they are a loan that must be paid back. If you don't pay your bill on time or in full when it's due, you will owe a finance charge. The finance charge depends on your outstanding balance and the annual percentage rate (APR). For example, if your card carries an

18% interest rate and you leave a balance of $100 on the card, it will cost you an extra $18 to pay off the balance the next month.

DEBIT CARD — A debit card allows you to make purchases in real-time by accessing your money from your checking or savings account electronically. If you have insufficient funds in your bank account, you will be charged an overdraft fee between $30-40 or more.

What is the Fine Print?

When applying for credit cards, it's important to shop around. Fees, interest rates, finance charges, and benefits can vary greatly. In some cases, credit cards seem like great deals until you read the fine print and disclosures. When you're trying to find the credit card that's right for you, look at the:

ANNUAL PERCENTAGE RATE (APR) — The APR measures the cost of credit, in terms of a yearly interest rate. It must be disclosed before your account can be activated, and it must appear on your account statements. The credit card issuer also must disclose the "periodic rate" — the rate applied to your outstanding balance to figure the finance charge for each billing period.

Some credit card plans allow the issuer to change your APR when interest rates or other economic indicators, called indexes, change. Because the rate change is linked to the index's performance, these plans are called "variable rate" programs. Rate changes raise or lower the finance charge on your account. If you're considering a variable rate card, the issuer also must tell you that the rate may change and how the rate is determined. Before you become obligated on the account, you also must receive information about any limits on how much and how often your rate may change.

GRACE PERIOD — The grace period is the number of days you have to pay your bill in full without triggering a finance charge. For example, the credit card company may say that you have 25 days from the statement date, provided you paid your previous balance in full by the due date. The statement date is on the bill. The grace period usually applies only to new purchases. Most credit cards do not give a grace period for cash advances and balance transfers. Instead, interest charges start right away. If your card includes a grace period, the issuer must mail your bill at least 14 days before the due date so you'll have enough time to pay.

ANNUAL FEES — Many issuers charge annual membership or participation fees. Some card issuers assess the fee in monthly installments.

TRANSACTION FEES AND OTHER CHARGES — Some issuers charge a fee if you use the card to get a cash advance, make a late payment, or exceed your credit limit. Some charge a monthly fee if you use the card — or if you don't.

CUSTOMER SERVICE — Customer service is something most people don't consider, or appreciate, until there's a problem. Look for a 24-hour toll-free telephone number.

UNAUTHORIZED CHARGES — If your card is used without your permission, you can be held responsible for up to $50 per card. If you report the loss before the card is used, you can't be held responsible for any unauthorized charges. To minimize your liability, report the loss as soon as possible. Some issuers have 24-hour toll-free telephone numbers to accept emergency information. It's a good idea to follow-up with a letter to the issuer, include your account number, the date you noticed your card missing, and the date you reported the loss. Keep a record, in a safe place separate from your cards, of your account numbers, expiration dates, and the telephone numbers of each card issuer so you can report a loss quickly.

Alternatives to Borrowing

Before seeking a student loan, explore other ways to pay for your college education. Here are some ideas:

- ✓ Check with CCSU's Scholarship Office. Look first for funds that you do not have to pay back. Some scholarships are based on need, some on academic merit, on test scores, athletic skill, musical or artistic talent, community or volunteer, activities, or other special abilities.
- ✓ Investigate awards offered by religious groups, fraternal organizations, or civic groups.
- ✓ Check with employers and organizations connected with your field of interest for scholarship opportunities.
- ✓ Search for outside scholarship using **www.fastweb.com** and **www.finaid.org**
- ✓ Consider student employment. Financial Aid may find you eligible for Federal Work-Study (FWS), the Career Services department maintains a list of available work student positions on College Central Network **www.collegecentral.com/ccsu/**
- ✓ Career Services is another source of part-time jobs is the Career Services department maintains a list of available on campus and off campus jobs, available on College Central Network
- ✓ Consider working summers and holidays to help pay tuition and expenses

Student Loans

If all other alternatives have been explored, education loans can be an excellent way for students to pay educational expenses; however, the debt should be considered carefully. Student loans are a serious financial obligation that you must repay. Borrowing to pay for college has long term implications as the amount of money you borrow can seriously affect your life after you leave school. You will want to carefully consider the career choice you have made in relation to the amount you borrow. Some professions offer low to moderate level salaries which make it difficult for you to pay sizable loan payments.

In addition to the amount you borrow, all student loans will charge you interest. This interest is often lower than that for other types of loans and payment on the loan is deferred until about 6–9 months after you leave school. Your loan repayment, or lack of repayment, will affect your credit rating and ability to borrow for other purposes, such as a car or house. Timely repayment builds your credit rating. An inability to pay your loan, may result in additional late charges, collection costs, court cost and attorney fees as well as developing a poor credit rating. If you decide a loan is consider the following:

- ✓ **AMOUNT OF LOAN:** Think about how much you need to borrow. You may not want to borrow the full amount for which you are eligible.
- ✓ **NUMBER OF LOANS:** Your plans for further study will affect your total indebtedness. For example, are you going to graduate school?
- ✓ **LOAN LIMITS:** Most loan programs specify minimum and maximum amounts you can borrow.
- ✓ **REPAYMENT:** You can avoid multiple monthly payments by, when possible, staying with one loan program.
- ✓ **LENGTH OF REPAYMENT PERIOD:** You will save interest costs if you choose a shorter repayment period (although monthly payments will be higher). Federal Stafford Loans offer a variety of repayment options.

All student loans are considered federal direct subsidized or unsubsidized loans. A subsidized loan is based off need and the interest is paid for by the government while you are in school. Unsubsidized loans are not need-based and the borrower (student or guardian) is responsible for the interest but doesn't have to pay it until the student is out of school.

INTEREST RATES FOR DIRECT LOANS FIRST DISBURSED ON OR AFTER JULY 1, 2017

Loan Type	Borrower Type	Loans first disbursed on or after 7/1/17 and before 7/1/18	Loans first disbursed on or after 7/1/16 and before 7/1/17
Federal Direct Subsidized Loans	Undergraduate	4.45%	3.76%
Federal Direct Unsubsidized Loans	Undergraduate	4.45%	3.76%
Federal Direct Unsubsidized Loans	Graduate or Professional	6.00%	5.31%
Federal Direct PLUS Loans	Parents and Graduate or Professional Students	7.00%	6.31%

MINIMUM MONTHLY PAYMENTS: Monthly payments will depend on the amount you borrow, and the repayment plan you select.

BORROWERS RIGHTS AND RESPONSIBILITIES: Be sure you understand your rights and responsibilities under each loan program. The school gives you these. Keep all paperwork for future reference.

HOW MUCH WILL YOU BE ABLE TO "PAY LATER"?: To decide how much indebtedness, you can probably manage when you graduate, consider your expected starting salary, earnings prospects and your lifestyle. Then, estimate your anticipated level of debt and monthly payments and see if the two are in the same range. If you cannot afford your projected payments, then try to borrow less. Try to be realistic when projecting your future earnings and the amount you will need to pay living expenses after graduation. Remember, starting a new job and setting up living arrangements will require extra resources and create a heavy initial demand on your new income. You can review the median pay for occupations in the U.S. Bureau of Labor Statistics' Occupational Outlook Handbook at **www.bls.gov/ooh.**

SAMPLE REPAYMENT SCHEDULE

Loan Type	Amount Borrowed	Interest Rate	Monthly Payment	Total Interest	Total Paid	Months
Federal Stafford	$3,000.00	8.25%	$50.00	$874.00	$3,874.00	76
Federal Stafford	$5,000.00	8.25%	$61.00	$2,359.00	$7,359.00	120
Federal Stafford	$15,000.00	8.25%	$184.00	$7,078.00	$22,078.00	120

Your Exit Interview

About two months before the end of your last semester at the university, you will receive a notice that you need to complete an Exit Interview if you have received a Federal Direct Student Loan. During the interview, you will receive information about repaying your loans. Most loans have a "grace" period of six or nine months. You do not have to start repayment for this length of time after you graduate, withdraw or enroll for less than half time. Refer to your promissory note copy for this length of time. If you can make payments on your loan during your grace period, do so. Grace period payments are interest-free and can greatly reduce the overall amount of interest you pay. For more information, go to **https://studentloans.gov**

Loan Repayment

When your federal direct loan is due you will hear from the federal servicer. If you do not hear from someone regarding your loan within 60 days of leaving CCSU, call your federal servicer. When you signed your promissory note, you agreed to contact your servicer when you leave school.

Federal Consolidation Loans

Consolidation Loans allow you to combine certain federal student loans. It allows you to make one monthly payment rather than multiple payments to various lenders. If you borrow money each year, you will have more than one loan; they are not extensions of one loan. You can consolidate these multiple loans into one and pay a lower interest rate. However, consolidation may result in the loss of deferment benefits. You may wish to speak with a member of the Financial Aid Office before making this decision. If you have both Stafford Loans and a William D. Ford Direct Loan, you can consolidate through the federal government by calling Direct Loan Consolidation at 1-800-557-7392. There is no charge for consolidating your loans.

Good Credit Records

For most students, a student loan is the first experience with credit. Student loans can be an excellent way to establish a good credit rating. Pay your student loan promptly each month. Frequent late payments constitute delinquency and may harm your credit history. Here are some tips on establishing good credit:

- ✓ Notify the necessary parties regarding change of address or name change. Federal Direct Loan changes should be referred to the servicing agent which is on the loan statement.
- ✓ Send the payment due each month, even if you haven't received a bill. When you can, send extra payments to reduce your total interest.
- ✓ Always call the appropriate servicing agent if you have a question or problem.
- ✓ Never ignore correspondence or a payment request.

Loan Rehabilitation

If you default on your NDSL or Federal Perkins Loan, you may rehabilitate your defaulted loan by requesting the rehabilitation and by making an on-time, monthly payment, as determined by the loan holder, each month for twelve consecutive months. If you successfully rehabilitate your defaulted NDSL or Federal Perkins Loan, you will again be subject to the terms and conditions and qualify for the benefits and privileges of your original promissory note and the default will be removed from your credit history. You can rehabilitate a defaulted NDSL or Federal Perkins Loan only once.

Student Loan Ombudsman

If you find yourself in a situation where you are in a disagreement with the servicing agent and have not been able to resolve it yourself, you may need the assistance of an independent individual who can help rectify the situation. This person is called a Federal Student Assistance Student Loan Ombudsman of the Department of Education. The Student Loan Ombudsman will review and attempt to informally resolve your dispute and may be reached at 1-877-557-2575.

Activity #4: Financial Advice from your Elders

Ask a parent/guardian/grandparent/ other adult/ if they have any "lessons learned" regarding any topic discussed in this chapter including, but not limited to: financial budgeting, financial literacy, loans, investing, credit cards, credit scores, saving, etc.

1. What did this person say they wish they knew more about at your age?
2. Did they give you any helpful advice?
3. What were some lessons they learned from their past that might help you in the future?

Financial Protection

You wouldn't consider carrying around your cell phone without a protective case; the same should be true about protecting your financial information and investments.

Scams and Identity Theft

According to the web site of the Federal Trade Commission, personal information can be obtained from yearbook publishers, companies that make class rings or photograph school portraits, a driver's license, magazine subscriptions, book clubs, SAT preparation firms, formal wear companies that outfit students for their school proms, student directories, or any other activities that supply names, addresses and ages to companies who can make lucrative profits by selling the information.

If you are contacted by someone claiming to be from the Department of Education and you are offered a grant and asked for your bank account information, you should follow the outline below. The Department of Education suggests if you are the victim of this scam, you should take the following 4 steps:

1) Immediately contact your bank, explain the situation, and request that the bank monitor or close the compromised account.
2) Report the fraud to ED's Office of Inspector General hotline at 1-800-MIS-USED (1-800-647-8733) or **oig.hotline@ed.gov.** Special agents in the Office of Inspector General investigate fraud involving federal education dollars.
3) Report the fraud to the Federal Trade Commission (FTC). The FTC has an online complaint form at **www.ftc.gov,** hotline at 1-877-FTC-HELP (1-877-382-4357; teletype for the hearing impaired: 1-866-653-4261). The FTC will investigate if the fraud is deemed widespread; therefore, it is important that every student contacted by the person or people in question lodge a complaint so the FTC has an accurate idea of how many incidents have occurred. The FTC also has an Identity Theft Complaint Form and a Scholarship Scam Page at **www.consumer.ftc.gov/financialaid.**
4) Notify the police about the incident. Impersonating a federal officer is a crime, as is identity theft. When filing complaints, you should provide detailed information about the incident, including what was said, the name of the person who called, and from what number the call originated (if you were able to obtain it via Caller ID). Additionally, if unauthorized debits have already appeared against your bank account, you should mention this fact in your complaint. Records of such debits could be useful in locating the wrongdoer.

What is Phishing?

Phishing is a fraudulent, spoofed e-mail that looks like someone you do business with sent it. It will usually include official logos and look very authentic. The body of a Phishing e-mail may contain a message requesting that you update, validate, or verify your personal/Privacy Act protected information. The purpose of the e-mail is to get you to disclose personal/Privacy Act protected information such as PINs, social security numbers, account numbers, mother's maiden name, passwords, etc. Some e-mail may also contain links that take you to an "official looking" web site that set up a scenario in which personal/Privacy Act protected information is requested. These web sites may not be legitimate!

Protecting Against Phishing E-mails

To minimize risk to yourself, if you receive Phishing e-mail:

- ✓ Never give out personally identifiable information in an e-mail or to a web site that has a link in an e-mail without validating it with the legitimate source.
- ✓ Do not open email with attachments or enclosures if they are from unknown sources.
- ✓ Do not reply to the e-mail.
- ✓ Do not type or paste any information into the e-mail.
- ✓ Do not click on any links contained within the e-mail from any unknown source.
- ✓ Use an open source tool. There are many commercial as well as free open source tools that con protect one from Phishing. A web search for "spoof guard," "Phishing protection," and "password hashing security" will reveal many of these tools. SpoofGuard and Netcraft Toolbar are only examples of the products available.

What is Pharming?

Pharming is the next generation of e-mail phishing attacks. However, it is not spoofing an email, it is a URL that redirects you to a fraudulent URL without your knowledge. There are several methods the pharmer uses to accomplish this, all of which are very hard to detect. You might type a valid URL in your browser only to end up at a fraudulent site that looks just like the one you thought you were going to access.

Protecting Against Pharming

To minimize risk to yourself, if you receive a Pharming URL:

- ✓ Use anti-virus software and a firewall. AVG and Zonealarm are examples of products available.
- ✓ Ensure that your browser is kept up to date and security patches are applied.
- ✓ Install a spyware detection and removal program. Ad-aware is only one example of the numerous products available to the public.
- ✓ Consider installing a Web browser tool bar to help protect from known fraud websites. IE 7 and Netcraft Toolbar are examples of the products available.
- ✓ Look for website privacy policies. Avoid doing business with any site that does not post its privacy policy.
- ✓ Limit the number of websites and amount of personal information you share on the Internet.
- ✓ Look for misspelled words and bad formatting. This may be an indication of a pharming site.
- ✓ If a password is needed, enter an incorrect password first.
- ✓ Use a reputable Internet Service Provider.

Emergency Funding and Assistance at CCSU

Unexpected circumstances can result in difficult and sometimes extreme financial situations. If you find yourself having to live in your car or choosing between food or gas/bus fare to get to class - caring individuals at the university want to know and can help you. You may need to set pride aside in order to get back on your feet. Reach out to someone at Student Affairs, the Financial Aid Office, a Professor, Coach, Department Advisor, Department Chair, Dean, or other university personnel you trust.

Some emergency fund money is not advertised. If you are struggling and cannot afford books, clothing, certification fees etc., speak to a professor or department chair. These individuals can help connect you with university emergency applications.

There is food bank, called Maria's Place on campus.

- ✓ This is a FREE service for all current CCSU students, faculty, and staff who are in need of food assistance.
- ✓ During the first visit you will need to present your CCSU Bluechip Card.
- ✓ A volunteer will guide you through the process for future visits.
- ✓ Those using the pantry may take TEN items of food per visit
- ✓ Please bring grocery bags
- ✓ Visits to the pantry are confidential and volunteers will maintain privacy

In conclusion, whether you have a limited or significant income, if you don't budget properly you can find yourself falling short of your goals. Set clear goals and then plan a budget that will take care of the necessities and allow you to save so that you can reach your long-term goals of independence, and perhaps things like owning a home, traveling etc. Save, even if it is only a very small amount – the habit is key to financial success. Good budgeting will also allow you to build a good credit score which again will aid you with future.

Chapter Summary

- ✓ Financial Literacy refers to the set of skills and knowledge that allows an individual to make informed and effective decisions with all of their financial resources.
- ✓ The Career Success Center at CCSU can assist you in finding work on campus, discipline-related internships, and career employment after graduation.
- ✓ Whether you have a limited or significant income, if you don't budget properly you can find yourself falling short of your goals.

- ✓ Check your credit score at least once per year to prevent fraud and check for accuracy.
- ✓ Educate yourself on all your options for financial aid. Including grants, scholarships, and the different types of loans (be aware of the differences between loan types).
- ✓ Student loans are a serious financial obligation that you must repay. Borrowing to pay for college has long term implications as the amount of money you borrow can seriously affect your life after you leave school.
- ✓ Set clear goals and then plan a budget that will take care of the necessities and allow you to save so you can reach your long-term goals of independence, and perhaps things like owning a home, traveling etc.
- ✓ According to the web site of the Federal Trade Commission, personal information can be obtained from not only a driver's license but magazine subscriptions, yearbook publishers, and any companies who sell your information, such as your name and address.

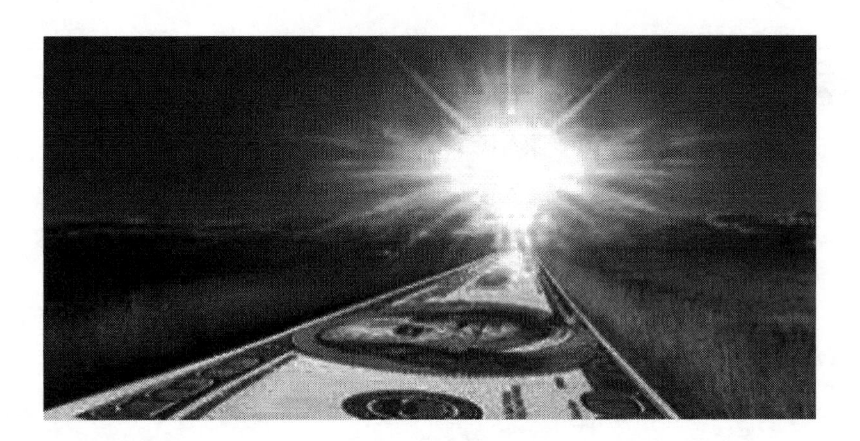

Chapter Review Questions

1) What does it mean to have financial wellness?
2) What are the 5 components of financial literacy?
3) How are earnings and spending related?
4) What is the difference between a "need" and a "want"?
5) What criteria are used to produce a credit report and credit score?
6) Why is a good credit score important?
7) If you don't pay off a credit card in full each month, what fees will you incur?
8) What is the guideline for how much debt compared to earnings?
9) What does "Pay yourself first" mean?
10) What are some things to consider when borrowing money?
11) How are student loans different from regular loans?
12) How can you protect yourself against fraud, phishing, pharming, and identity theft?
13) Where can you go on campus to find financial assistance?

Website Resources

CAREER AND SALARY PLANNING SITES

- ✓ Salary: **www.salary.com**
- ✓ U.S. Department of Labor Bureau of Labor Statistics: **www.bls.gov/ncs/ocs/compub.htm**
- ✓ U.S. Bureau of Labor Statistics, Occupational Outlook Handbook: **www.bls.gov/ooh**
- ✓ College Grad: **www.collegegrad.com**

CREDIT

- ✓ Money and Credit: **www.consumer.ftc.gov/topics/money-credit**
- ✓ Credit and loans: **www.consumer.ftc.gov/topics/credit-and-loans**
- ✓ View credit reports from each of the three big credit agencies (Equifax, Transunion, and Experian) for free: www.annualcreditreport.com or **www.creditkarma.com**
- ✓ Gift Cards: **www.consumer.ftc.gov/articles/0182-gift-cards**

FINANCIAL LITERACY WEB SITES:

- ✓ JumpStart Coalition: **www.jumpstart.org**
- ✓ Kiplinger: **www.kiplinger.com**
- ✓ National Endowment for Financial Education (NEFE): **www.nefe.org**
- ✓ Stretcher (How to stretch your money) **www.stretcher.com**
- ✓ 360 Degrees of Financial Literacy: **www.360financialliteracy.org**
    - Offers finance information for different life stages and personal situations.
- ✓ Smart About Money: **www.smartaboutmoney.org**
    - Provides online resources, calculators, and other information and tools on a wide range of money topics, including daily decision-making, emergencies, debt management, life transitions, and work and money.
- ✓ MyMoney.Gov: **www.mymoney.gov**
    - Five key money topics: earn, save and invest, protect, spend, and borrow: **www.mymoney.gov**

FINANCIAL TERMS

- ✓ Banking Terms and Phrases: **www.helpwithmybank.gov/dictionary/index-dictionary.html**
- ✓ Credit Card Contract Definitions: **www.consumerfinance.gov/data-research/credit-card-data/know-you-owe-credit-cards/credit-card-contract-definitions/**
- ✓ Student Loan Glossary: **www.fastweb.com/financial-aid/articles/student-loan-glossary**

LOAN INFORMATION

- ✓ Comparing Federal and Private Student Loans (1-page PDF comparison chart); **www.studentaid.ed.gov/sa/sites/default/files/federal-vs-private-loans-graphic.pdf**

PROTECTION

- ✓ Identity Theft Prevention: **www.ed.gov/misused**
- ✓ Last Pass (Identify theft prevention); Stores passwords: **www.lastpass.com**
- ✓ Financial Aid Scam Prevention: **www.studentaid.ed.gov/lsa**

- ✓ Scholarship Scam Prevention: **www.ftc.consumer.gov/financialaid**
- ✓ Consumer Financial Protection Bureau (CFPB): **www.consumerfinance.gov**
- ✓ U.S. Department of Education: legitimate information on scholarships, financial assistance, federal student aid: **www.studentaid.ed.gov** (800) 433-3243
- ✓ Better Business Bureau (reliability of companies): **www.bbb.org**
- ✓ Federal Trade Commission (FTC) monitors financial aid fraud: **www.ftc.gov** (English), **www.ftc.gov/es** (Spanish), consumer help line: (877) 382-4357

Interactive Financial Literacy and Money Management Websites

These websites provide a variety of tools to learn financial budgeting, salary calculations, how to handle debt, and making wise choices to save money, etc.

- ✓ What Are the Four Life Values? (course) **www.smartaboutmoney.org**
- ✓ Life Values Quiz: **www.smartaboutmoney.org**
- ✓ Money Personality Quiz: **www.moneyharmonyymoney.com**
- ✓ 30-Steps to Financial Wellness: **www.financialliteracymonth.com/30steps**
- ✓ Managing Money during College: **www.studentaid.ed.gov**
- ✓ Cash course: Your Real-Life Money Guide: **www.cashcourse.org**
- ✓ IGrad: Financial Literacy and Career Resources: **www.igrad.com**
- ✓ Salary Calculator: **www.jobsearchintelligence.com/etc/jobseekers/salary-calculator.php**
- ✓ Cost of Living Calculator: **www.nerdwallet.com/cost-of-living-calculator**
- ✓ FlexScore: **www.flexscore.com**
- ✓ NextAdvisor: **www.nextadvsior.com**
- ✓ Spendster: **www.spendster.com/tools**
- ✓ Khan Academy Better Money Habits: **www.bettermoneyhabits.com**

References

www.financialeducatorscouncil.org/financial-literacy-definition, retrieved 2017

Chapter 9

Disease Risks and Illness Awareness

By Matthew Orange, PhD, Kathy Pirog, MS, ATC, Thomas McCarthy, MS, ATC and Peter Morano, PhD, ATC

Chapter Objectives

After reading this chapter, students should be able to:

- ✓ Define cardiovascular disease and describe its risk factors;
- ✓ Define cancer, explain the role of heritance and environmental factors to its cause, and recognize its incidence and the number of deaths it causes each year;
- ✓ Define community-based diseases and list common "touch surfaces" that contribute to their spread;
- ✓ Discuss best practices for preventing the spread of community-based diseases, including good personal hygiene habits, good laundering and housekeeping habits, and basic habits of good health;
- ✓ Describe signs/symptoms, and prevention of the most common types of pathogens; blood borne pathogens; common fungal and parasitic infections;
- ✓ Discuss risk factors of sexually transmitted infections; and
- ✓ Explain basic concepts of CPR and First Aid.

Disease Risk and Awareness

"He who cures a disease may be the skillfullest,
but he that prevents is the safest physician" - Thomas Fuller

Diseases that impact our physical being (as opposed to our mental or psychological state) can be separated into two main types – chronic disease and infectious disease. A chronic disease is one that takes a long time to develop and is quite often linked to lifestyle behaviors. Risk of developing chronic diseases such as heart disease, most cancers, and type II diabetes increases as a result of poor diet, sedentary lifestyles, and the use of tobacco or other drugs. Infectious diseases result from contracting a pathogen (viral or bacterial) from another human, insects, animals, or from food. Symptoms of infectious diseases can manifest themselves within hours or months after contracting the pathogen (in the case of HIV, it could take years). Examples of viral infections are the common cold, the flu, herpes, chicken pox, and HIV. Examples of bacterial infections are strep throat, chlamydia, salmonella, and urinary tract infections.

Chronic disease typically requires extensive interventions and treatment that can last the rest of a person's life. A change to one's lifestyle is often needed to successfully combat chronic disease (quitting smoking, improving diet, exercising, etc.). Bacterial infections can often be treated and cured by the use of antibiotics. Viral infections however, often have no cure but are treatable and managed with the use of medications. Vaccines are available for many viral and bacterial infections, which drastically reduce the chance of contraction.

In this chapter, we will specifically discuss the chronic diseases that have the largest impact on health and wellness in the United States, cardiovascular disease and cancer. As part of our discussions, we will address the risk factors for these diseases and consider strategies to limit our own personal risk. We will then discuss best practices for prevention of infectious diseases, and, finally, we will consider the basics of first aid and CPR. It should be noted that much of our current understanding of disease prevalence, the risk factors that contribute to their progression, and the mechanisms by which infectious diseases are spread is due to the work of epidemiologists. These scientists investigate the occurrence and spread of disease in an attempt to influence public health by way of disease prevention.

Cardiovascular Disease

Cardiovascular disease (CVD) is an encompassing term meaning a disease of the heart and blood vessels (What is Cardiovascular Disease, 2017). Several specific conditions are comprised under the umbrella of CVD including coronary heart disease (CHD) and stroke which are the #1 and #5 killers of Americans, respectively. Also, within CVD is hypertension and high cholesterol which are not only conditions in and of themselves, but also risk factors for CHD and stroke.

Coronary heart disease (CHD) is a chronic condition that is the result of a waxy substance called plaque that builds up inside the coronary arteries and is the #1 killer of Americans. The clogging of these vessels is called atherosclerosis, which occurs over many years. If the flow of oxygen to the heart is slowed or blocked, angina pectoris or a heart attack can occur (What is Coronary Artery Disease, 2017). Hypertension, or high blood pressure, is often termed the "silent killer" because people do not feel or notice when they have it until they experience a major medical event. Hypertension occurs when the pressure blood in the vessels is higher than it should be (High Blood Pressure, 2017). If your arteries have plaque build-up (atherosclerosis), or if the arteries become hardened (arteriosclerosis) then the pressure inside the arteries will increase.

A stroke is a disruption of blood flow to the brain. The blood flow disruption can be from a blocked artery in the brain (ischemic stroke) or if an artery in the brain leaks or ruptures (hemorrhagic stroke). Ischemic strokes are the most common, accounting for 87% of all strokes. A third type of stroke is a transient ischemic attack, or a ministroke. This occurs when there is a temporary artery blockage and is considered a warning sign of a future stroke. Even though a TIA is not a full-blown stroke and there is rarely lasting impairment, it is still a medical emergency and 911 should be called (American Stroke Association, 2017).

Cholesterol is a fatty substance that travels in the blood on proteins called lipoproteins. Our body makes its own cholesterol, but we also get some through our diet. There are 2 types of cholesterol – high density lipoproteins (HDL) and low-density lipoproteins (LDL). The HDL cholesterol is a healthy type of cholesterol and actually protects against CVD. The LDL cholesterol is unhealthy and increases the risk of CVD. LDL cholesterol can build up on the inside of your arteries causing blood flow to be reduced or blocked. This cholesterol build-up can occur in the heart causing heart disease or a heart attack. Triglycerides are another type of fatty substance that circulates in the blood. High triglyceride levels also increase risk of heart disease (High Blood Cholesterol, 2017).

Risk Factors for Cardiovascular Disease

Many of the factors that can increase the risk of any form of CVD can be attributed to lifestyle behaviors. The following are primary risk factors for CVD. All of the primary risk factors are controllable, meaning we can actively take steps to reduce the risk from these factors (What is Cardiovascular Disease, 2017).

- ✓ Smoking
- ✓ Lack of physical activity
- ✓ Unhealthy diet
- ✓ High cholesterol
- ✓ Hypertension
- ✓ Obesity
- ✓ Diabetes
- ✓ Stress

If we smoke, eat a poor diet or do not exercise, we are making a choice to do those things. We may not choose to have high blood pressure or cholesterol, but we can choose to manage those conditions. Other factors that can contribute to the risk of CVD are:

- ✓ Age
- ✓ Heredity
- ✓ Excessive alcohol consumption

Activity #1: CVD Risk Factors

Let's Reflect!

- ✓ How many risk factors of CVD do you have?
- ✓ Are the risk factors that you have controllable?
- ✓ If yes, what steps can you take to minimize your risk? (i.e. begin to start eating a healthier diet and exercise 3 times a week)

Signs and Symptoms of Cardiovascular Disease

If you are exhibiting any of the risk factors now, you are laying a groundwork for CVD. When someone is having a heart attack, they will often exhibit some signs or symptoms (Figure 1). However, the signs or symptoms could be mild enough that the person experiencing them may not even realize they are having a heart attack, or the victim may think the signs/symptoms are unrelated to a cardiac event (food poisoning, indigestion, flu-like symptoms). Ignoring the possibility of a heart attack could lead to a delay in seeking medical help. This is of particular concern in middle-aged individuals who exhibit one or more of the primary risk factors.

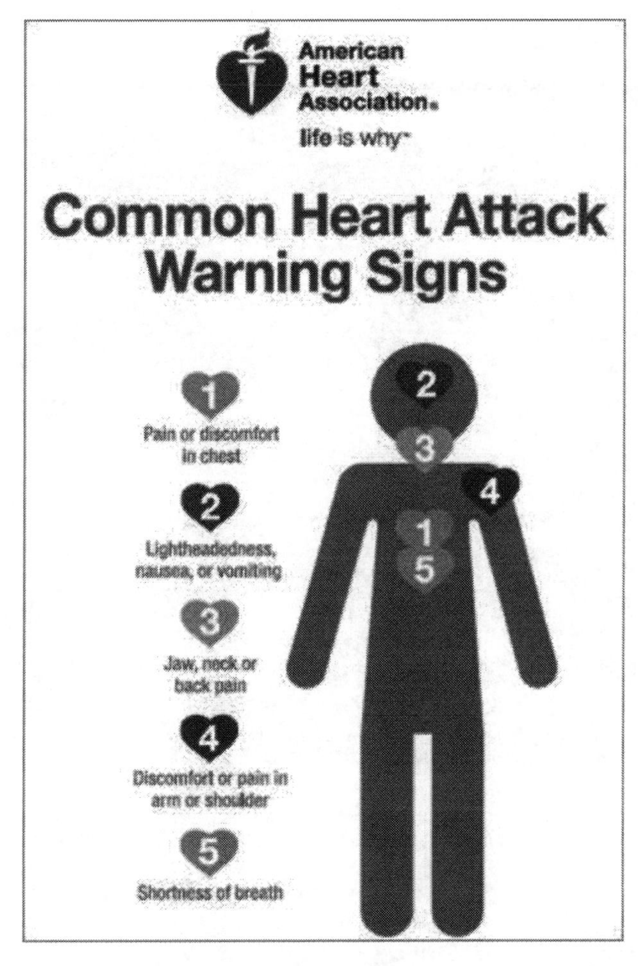

Figure 1. Common Heart Attack Warning Signs

Hypertension can be prevented through healthy lifestyle behaviors and it can be treated with medication and exercise. Since there are rarely any signs or symptoms for high blood pressure, the best thing you can do is make sure you know your blood pressure from annual medical check-ups. Normal blood pressure is around 120/80 mm/Hg. The top number is the systolic pressure or the pressure in the arteries during a heartbeat. The bottom number is the diastolic pressure or the pressure in the arteries between heartbeats. Table 1 outlines categories of blood pressure.

Table 1. Blood Pressure Categories

BLOOD PRESSURE CATEGORY	SYSTOLIC mm Hg (upper number)		DIASTOLIC mm Hg (lower number)
NORMAL	LESS THAN 120	and	LESS THAN 80
ELEVATED	120 – 129	and	LESS THAN 80
HIGH BLOOD PRESSURE (HYPERTENSION) STAGE 1	130 – 139	or	80 – 89
HIGH BLOOD PRESSURE (HYPERTENSION) STAGE 2	140 OR HIGHER	or	90 OR HIGHER
HYPERTENSIVE CRISIS (consult your doctor immediately)	HIGHER THAN 180	and/or	HIGHER THAN 1

People with unmanaged high blood pressure are of particular risk for stroke. There are distinct signs and symptoms for a stroke that often suddenly appear (Figure 2). If any of them appear present, call 911 immediately.

- ✓ Numbness on one side of the body (face, arm, leg) often accompanied by sagging in the face
- ✓ Confusion, trouble speaking or understanding
- ✓ Difficulty seeing
- ✓ Trouble walking, loss of balance, dizziness or lack of coordination
- ✓ Severe headache

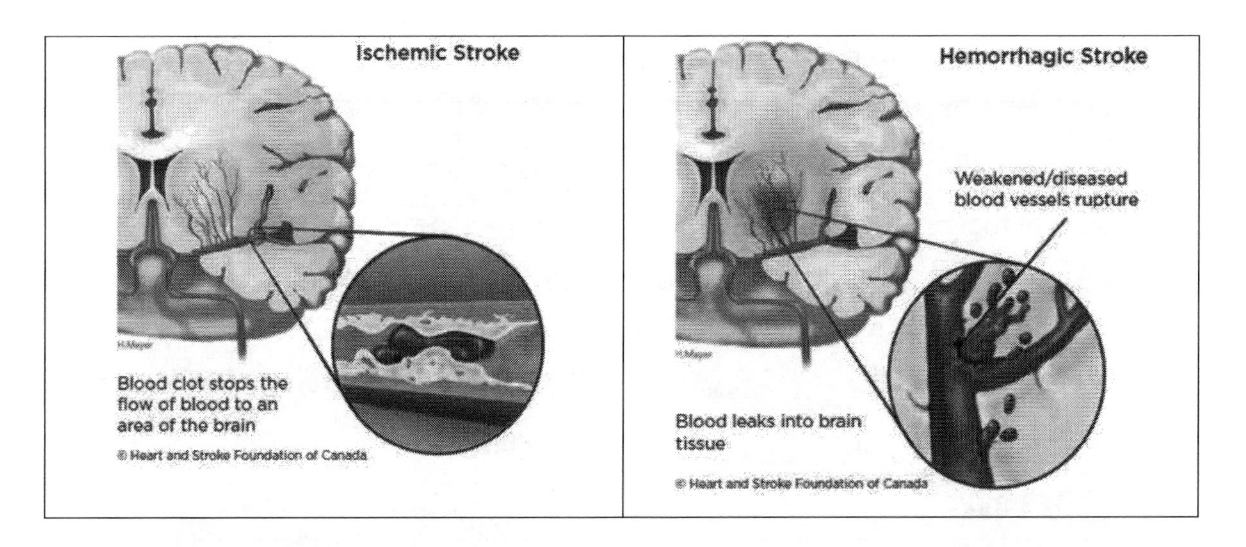

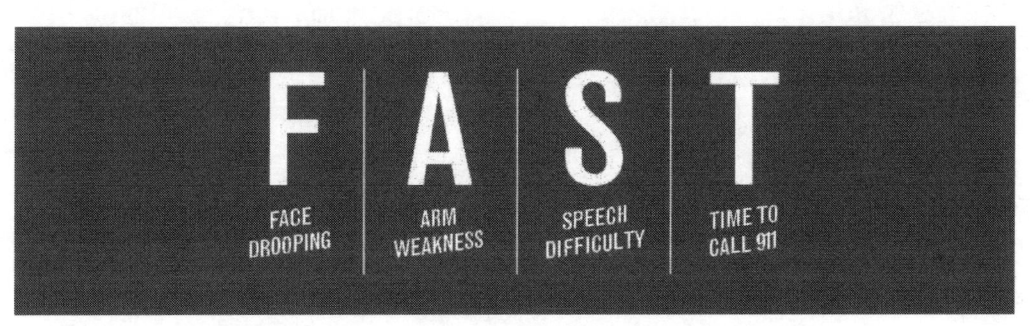

Figure 2. Signs and Symptoms of a Stroke

Since there are no signs or symptoms of having high cholesterol/triglycerides, knowing your cholesterol and triglyceride levels is the first step in reducing the risk it may pose on your health. These levels can be checked through a blood test when you have a physical check-up by your primary care physician. When examining blood cholesterol, there are several things to consider - the first is total cholesterol levels. It is recommended that total cholesterol be under 200mg/dL (milligrams per deciliter). The second consideration is the amounts of cholesterol for each type: LDL should be under 100mg/dL and HDL should be above 40mg/dL. The third consideration is your cholesterol ration. To calculate this, divide your total cholesterol by your HDL levels (High Blood Cholesterol, 2017). The optimal value should be 4 or less. Triglyceride levels should be below 150mg/dL. Table 2 outlines categories for blood cholesterol.

Table 2. Blood Cholesterol Categories

TOTAL CHOLESTEROL LEVEL	HEALTH CATEGORY
Less than 200 mg/dL	Desirable
200-239 mg/dL	Borderline High
240 mg/dL and above	High

Source: High Blood Cholesterol, 2017

LDL CHOLESTEROL LEVEL	LDL CHOLESTEROL CATEGORY
Less than 100 mg/dL	Optimal
100-129 mg/dL	Near Optimal/above average
130-159 mg/dL	Borderline High
160-189 mg/dL	High
190 mg/dL and above	Very High

Source: High Blood Cholesterol, 2017

Cancer

Cancer is a group of diseases characterized by uncontrolled division of abnormal cells that can invade neighboring tissue and disrupt bodily functions (Cancer Prevention and Control, 2017). Cancer is second only to heart disease in terms of the number of lives it claims each year in the United States. In 2016, over 1.6 million new cancer cases were diagnosed, and there were almost 600,000 cancer related deaths (Cancer Statistics, 2017). Lung cancer is the deadliest (causes the largest number of annual deaths), due in large part to late detection (Common Cancer Types, 2017). Skin cancer is the most common, due to the fact that people are more regularly exposed to sunlight than any other cancer-causing agent (Skin Cancer Facts & Statistics, 2017).

The underlying cause of any cancer is a genetic abnormality. That is, a gene mutation upsets the normal cell life cycle leading to uncontrolled cell proliferation. While family history, inherited genetic information, and age do contribute to cancer risk, many risk factors are environmental and/or behavioral, and thereby, controllable.

Risk Factors for Cancer

Age and family history are not factors that we can control, but much of cancer risk is connected to our surroundings and choices. Controllable sources of cancer risk are listed below (Risk Factors for Cancer, 2015).

- ✓ Alcohol consumption
- ✓ Chronic inflammation
- ✓ Diet
- ✓ Hormones
- ✓ Immunosuppression
- ✓ Infectious agents
- ✓ Obesity
- ✓ Radiation
- ✓ Tobacco use
- ✓ UV exposure (typically from sunlight, but also from tanning booths)
- ✓ Exposure to cancer-causing substances

Activity #2: Cancer Risk Factors

Let's Reflect!

- ✓ How many risk factors of Cancer do you have?
- ✓ Are these risk factors controllable?
- ✓ If yes, what steps can you take to minimize you risk?

Cancer-causing substances, or carcinogens, are found in many foods, industrial agents, etc. Exposure to a carcinogen does not guarantee that you will develop cancer, but it does increase risk. A list of some of the well-known carcinogens is listed below (Cancer-Causing Substances in the Environment, 2015).

- ✓ Arsenic
- ✓ Asbestos
- ✓ Benzene

- ✓ Cadmium
- ✓ Formaldehyde
- ✓ Emissions from coal combustion
- ✓ Mineral oils
- ✓ Radon
- ✓ Secondhand tobacco smoke
- ✓ Soot
- ✓ Wood dust

Limiting Your Cancer Risk

Now that we have a general idea of what things increase your risk of developing cancer, let us discuss what you can do to limit that risk. First, we should do everything in our power to avoid consuming or using carcinogens. Risk for cancer is particularly high for those that both smoke and consume alcohol. Do not smoke and limit, as much as possible, your alcohol consumption. While many in the United States choose to consume alcohol, despite the inherent risk, it is important to do so in moderation. Currently, moderate use is considered to be up to one drink per day in women, and up to two drinks per day in men (Alcohol & Cancer Risk, 2013).

Evidence to support that specific components of a diet may increase or decrease cancer risk is limited. However, since risk for developing specific cancers (breast, colorectal, prostate, and uterine cancers) increases with obesity, the Centers for Disease Control and Prevention (CDC) encourages maintenance of a healthy weight via physical activity and consumption of a healthy diet (Cancer Prevention & Control, 2017).

In terms of physical activity, the CDC recommends you perform 150 minutes of moderate-intensity and 75 minutes of vigorous exercise each week (Physical Activity for a Healthy Weight, 2015). CDC recommendations for a diet that will achieve a healthy weight are listed below:

- ✓ Your diet should be within your daily calorie needs.
- ✓ Your sources of proteins should be beans, eggs, fish, lean meats, poultry, and nuts.
- ✓ Your diet should prioritize fruits, milk products that are low-fat or fat-free, vegetables, and whole grains.
- ✓ Your diet should be low in added sugars, cholesterol, salt, saturated fats, and *trans* fats.

You should limit your exposure to sunlight and its damaging UV rays, and tanning booths should not be used. While some UV is needed to kick start the metabolic processes that generate the active form of vitamin D, UV is a mutagen. That is, UV damages the DNA in skin cells, which may result in a cancer-causing mutation. You should do everything you can to cover yourself when outside and/or use sunscreen – the higher the SPF, the better. Increased damage to the skin from tanning beds adds to the risk. Tanning beds are linked to over 419,000 cases of skin cancer per year (Skin Cancer Facts & Statistics, 2017).

Finally, since prevention will never be 100% effective you should perform self-examinations for breast and testicular cancer, and follow the recommended schedule for breast, cervical, colorectal, and prostate cancer check-ups. For more information on self-examinations and recommended screening guidelines, you should visit the relevant pages on MedlinePlus (the information site of the National Institute of Health) and the website for the American Cancer Society.

- ✓ Breast self-exam
- ✓ Testicular self-exam
- ✓ American Cancer Society Guidelines for the Early Detection of Cancer

Activity #3: Self-Exams and Screening

View the websites MedlinePlus and perform the self-exam to screen yourself for either breast cancer or testicular cancer.

Community-Based Diseases

A university campus is not immune to the spread of infectious disease that can be considered to be community-based. A pathogen is anything that produce disease. Community-based pathogens are infectious disorders that can expose members of a campus society to a variety of health consequences. Awareness of the diverse types of commonly associated community-based pathogens along with knowledge of preventative measures, the early recognition of signs and symptoms are the key strategies for minimizing exposure and spread of diseases. Globally, public health care concerns continue to grow as antibiotic resistant organisms, along with the emergence of new pathogens challenge infectious control medical professionals.

The types of community-based pathogens that can be directly associated with a university campus include viral, bacterial, fungal, and parasitic diseases. The arrival of each new semester brings a host of organisms from a multitude of locations throughout the state, region, nation, and world as students and faculty assemble on to the university community. It is normal and often harmless for organisms to live in and on our bodies. With that said, some organism creates and transmit disease under certain conditions. The most obvious source of transmission for many pathogens occurs from our hands and from contact with common "touch surfaces." The consequence of such transmission may include gastrointestinal, respiratory, and skin infections.

Viral type diseases, such as gastroenteritis and upper respiratory infections known as URI's (common cold), tend to come in cycles on a university campus. In fact, this close quarter learning and living community is an excellent site for the incubation of disease. The typical cycle for the development of new strains occur approximately every 4-6 weeks. With this awareness, it is important that the university student utilize good personal hygiene and housekeeping practices throughout the semester. University students should understand that common "touch surfaces" are a breeding ground for disease. Students should be vigilant and focus on good personal hygiene, housekeeping and laundry practices in order to prevent and minimize infection risks.

Common touch surfaces should be a main focus of cleaning and sanitation in household and community settings in order to prevent and minimize the infection risk. Common "touch surfaces" on a college campus include:

- ✓ Work stations, academic station, academic classroom furniture, laboratories, technology, and computer centers.
- ✓ Building structures, such as door handles, hand railings, dormitory living and gathering areas, shared bathrooms.
- ✓ Athletic, wellness and recreation facilities including weight rooms, associated locker rooms, and showering areas.
- ✓ Equipment and clothing issued for physical education, athletics, recreation and club sports, theater and musical groups, as well as clothing and protective equipment found in the sciences.
- ✓ Food services- trays, utensils, counters, food stations, dining tables and chairs. Personal "touch surfaces" include:
- ✓ cell phones
- ✓ technology devices
- ✓ remote controls
- ✓ computer keyboards/touchscreens
- ✓ clothing
- ✓ athletic equipment

Best Practices for Preventing Community-Based Pathogens

The common theme to preventing community-based pathogens is awareness and commitment to practicing good personal hygiene habits, good health habits, good laundering and good house-keeping methods by all members of the campus community. Personal Hygiene and domestic housekeeping cleaning of apartments, dorm rooms, classrooms are important in minimizing outbreaks of pathogenic diseases. Domestic choirs include cleaning of bathrooms, bedding, and clothing on a regular (daily/weekly) basis.

Good Personal Hygiene Habits

1) Wash your hands often with soap and water, especially after using the bathroom, or coughing, or blowing your nose.
2) Make oral hygiene a daily habit: brush twice a day with fluoride toothpaste and change your toothbrush every 3 to 4 months.
3) Wash your clothing.
4) Shower immediately after activities where you have direct skin contact with people or shared surfaces, such as after exercising at a health club.
5) Keep cuts and scrapes clean and covered with bandages or dressing until healed.
6) Do not share personal items- towels, washcloths, razors and clothing, including uniforms.
7) Limit use of loofah pads when bathing/showering. These pads can be an excellent breeding ground for bacteria to hide. When used aggressively to exfoliate the skin the bacteria on the sponge now has an entry source into the body. Loofah pads used for bathing/showering should be:
    a. Allowed to dry daily;
    b. Not used for a few days after shaving;
    c. Never used on face or genitals;
    d. Washed weekly and replaced every 3-4 weeks; and
    e. Never be shared

Activity #3: Personal Hygiene Checklist

Go through the list of good personal hygiene habits. For this activity check off each habit that you *always* engage in, or you can mentally check them off in your head.

- ✓ Wash your hands often with soap and water, especially after using the bathroom, or coughing, or blowing your nose.
- ✓ Make oral hygiene a daily habit: brush twice a day with fluoride toothpaste and change your toothbrush every 3 to 4 months.
- ✓ Wash your clothing.
- ✓ Shower immediately after activities where you have direct skin contact with people or shared surfaces, such as after exercising at a health club.
- ✓ Limit use of loofah pads when bathing/showering.
- ✓ Keep cuts and scrapes clean and covered with bandages or dressing until healed.
- ✓ Do not share personal items- towels, washcloths, razors and clothing, including uniforms.

Practice Good Laundering and Housekeeping Habits

Clean and disinfect frequently touched surfaces, such as doorknobs, especially if someone is sick. This will help prevent the spread of flu to your friends and family and back to you.

1) Clean and disinfect frequently touched surfaces at home, work, or school.
2) Pay attention to doorknobs, keyboards, cell phones, faucets, trash cans.
3) Wash your sheets, pillowcases, blankets, and towels (minimally weekly).
4) Wash used sheets, towels, and clothes with water and laundry detergent. Use a dryer to dry them completely.
5) Wash clothes according to manufacturer's instructions on the label. Clean your hands after touching dirty clothes.

6) Use appropriate products:
    a. Cleaners or detergents are products that are used to remove soil, dirt, dust, organic matter, and germs (like bacteria, viruses, and fungi).
    b. Sanitizers are used to reduce germs from surfaces, but not totally get rid of them. Sanitizers reduce the germs from surfaces to levels that are considered safe.
    c. Disinfectants are chemical products that destroy or inactivate germs and prevent them from growing.

Practice Good Health Habits

1) Eat Nutritious Foods: 5-7 servings of fruits and veggies.
2) Stay Hydrated: 8-10 glasses of water daily.
3) Plenty of Rest: 7-8 hours of sleep each night.
4) Be Physically Active - exercise 3-4 times per week.
5) Manage your Stress.

Practice Health Habits to Stop the Spread of Germs

1) Avoid close contact with individuals who are sick.
2) Avoid close contact, such as kissing, hugging, or sharing cups or eating utensils with people who are sick.
3) Stay home when you are sick.
4) Wash your hands often with soap and water for 20 seconds or alcohol-based rubs.
5) Use a tissue or your upper shirt sleeve, not your hands to cover your mouth and nose when coughing or sneezing.
6) Avoid touching your eyes, nose, or mouth.
7) Get a new toothbrush after an illness.
8) Do not share personal items- towels, washcloths, razors and clothing, including uniforms.

The Center for Disease Control (CDC) is an excellent resource for current trends in defining, recommending prevention methods, providing signs/symptoms, as well as treatment plans and need for medical referral for common university-based pathogens. The CDC has documented and identified outbreaks of the following common community based pathogenic diseases that should be on the radar of all university students.

Use of Antibiotics and Antibiotic Resistance

Antibiotics can be a lifesaving drug that is commonly prescribed in medicine and should only be used to manage bacterial infections. Taking antibiotics for viral infections such as the "common cold" will not cure the infection or help you feel better. Most sore throats, bronchitis, sinus infections, and ear infections are best managed with over-the-counter medicines to manage/comfort current signs and symptoms, rest, hydration, nutrition, and time.

Key points to keep in mind:

- ✓ Antibiotics are not effective against viral infections.
- ✓ Bacteria will inevitably find ways of resisting the antibiotics developed by humans.
- ✓ Use of antibiotics for viral infections in the long run cause more harm than good as it increases your risk to antibiotic-resistant infections later.
- ✓ Antibiotics kills the healthy bacteria found in your gut.
- ✓ The other major factor in the growth of antibiotic resistance is spread of the resistant strains of bacteria from person to person, or from the non-human sources in the environment.
- ✓ The use of antibiotics in food producing animals has created an increase in antibiotic-resistance infections in humans.

Viral Pathogens

HAND, FOOT AND MOUTH: a viral disease that is highly contagious, therefore avoidance of close contact with contagious individuals is a must.

Signs/Symptoms: Fever, mouth sores, skin rash on hands and feet.

Prevention: hand sanitizers, hand washing, clean touch surfaces, good housekeeping practices.

MONONUCLEOSIS: is a viral infection caused by the Epstein-Barr virus.

Signs/Symptoms: extreme fatigue, fever, sore throat, head and body aches, swollen lymph nodes in neck and arm pit, swollen liver or spleen, rash.

Prevention: protect yourself by not sharing drinks or personal items or kissing someone who is infected. Avoid contact and collision sports until you are fully recovered as strenuous activity and contact may rupture your spleen.

INFLUENZA: influenza viruses infect the nose, throat, and sometimes the lungs. The associated illness usually starts suddenly, and the severity can range from mild to severe.

Signs/Symptoms: Fever or feeling feverish/chills, cough, sore throat, runny or stuffy nose, muscle or body aches, headaches, fatigue, vomiting and diarrhea.

Prevention: annual flu vaccination, practice good hygiene and housekeeping habits.

UPPER RESPIRATORY INFECTION: More than 200 viruses can cause the "common cold". Infections spreads person to person through the air and from close personal contact. The common cold needs to run its course and most people recover in about 7-10 days. Over-the-counter medicines may help ease symptoms but will not make your cold go away any faster. Antibiotics do not work against these viruses and have no impact on recovery time. Rest and fluid remain the best treatment options for the common cold.

Signs/Symptoms: Sore throat, stuffy or runny nose, coughing, post-nasal drip (mucus dripping down your throat), watery eyes, mild headache, mild body aches with symptoms peaking within 2-3 days and lingering for up to 10-14 days.

Prevention: wash your hands often and avoid touching your face with unwashed hands. Follow good hygiene habits and practice good health habits when ill.

NOROVIRUS: highly contagious, spread quickly and easily. Virus may take up to 2 weeks to exit the body. Individuals are most contagious when actively sick.

Signs/Symptoms: abdominal cramping, nausea, vomiting, diarrhea, fever, headache, and body aches.

Prevention: practice good personal hygiene. Since viral sources can be linked to eating or drinking items that are contaminated, touch surfaces and objects, sharing of foods and utensils. Do not share food, drinks, utensils, drink containers, or athletic clothing. Cleanliness in kitchen areas, washing of laundry.

VIRAL MENINGOCOCCAL: Viral meningitis is the most common type of meningitis, an inflammation of the tissue that covers the brain and spinal cord. There is no specific treatment for viral meningitis and most individuals will get better on their own within 7 to 10 days.

Signs/Symptoms: fever, headache, stiff neck, sensitivity to bright light, sleepiness, nausea/vomiting, lack of appetite, lack of energy.

Prevention: There are no vaccines to protect against viral meningitis, follow good personal hygiene and housekeeping practices.

Bacterial Pathogens

BACTERIAL MENINGOCOCCAL: A bacterial infection that causes swelling of the membranes that cover the brain. Bacterial meningitis is very serious as it can lead to death or cause serious complications, such as brain damage, hearing loss, or learning disabilities.

Signs/Symptoms: sudden onset of fever, severe headache, and stiff neck, nausea, vomiting, sensitivity to light, altered mental status.

Prevention: Meningococcal vaccination.

STAPHYLOCOCCUS INFECTIONS AND MRSA: Staphylococcus Aureus (MRSA) is bacteria that is commonly referred to a "super bug" due to its developed resistance to all forms of penicillin. The staphylococcus bacteria are commonplace on a university campus. It is found on persons, equipment, common touch surfaces, in shared facilities, classroom, dormitories, athletic and recreation facilities, and places of gatherings.

When a Methicillin-Resistant Staphylococcus Aureus (MRSA) outbreak occurs on university campus it is referred to as Community Acquired Methicillin-Resistant Staphylococcus Aureus (CA-MRSA). These infections usually manifest as skin infections, such as pimples and boils. MRSA is highly contractible. MRSA infection risk can be increased when participating in activities or places that involve crowding, skin-to-skin contact, and shared equipment or supplies. Hence, students and athletes are known to be at higher risk for acquiring CA-MRSA. CA-MRSA is preventable in a college environment, if everyone educates themselves and follows the policies for the prevention of MRSA infection.

Everyone has staphylococcus bacteria on their bodies. The cleanest person can get a staph infection. Staph can rub off the skin of an infected person and onto the skin of another person when they have skin-to-skin contact. Staph from an infected person can also get onto a commonly shared item (towels) or surface, and then get onto the skin of the person who touches it next. A staph infection irrupts when the bacteria enters the body through an open wound. A source of entry can be open cuts, scrapes, as well it can occur from shaving.

A staph infection is diagnosed as MRSA by taking a sample from the infected wound (either a small biopsy of skin or pus taken with a swab). The bacteria sample is cultured in a microbiology laboratory and tested to determine which antibiotics will be effective for treating the infection. Remember a staph infection may look "As Simple as a Pimple". Most Staph infections, including MRSA appear as a bump and it is common to think it is a spider bite. Unless the spider is seen, the irritation is not a spider bite, but rather the initial signs of a staph infection.

> Signs/Symptoms: Pus-filled abscess, drainage, redness, painful, swollen, warmth to surrounding tissue, fever, tender lymph nodes.
> Prevention: Practicing good personal hygiene habits, good health habits, good laundering and good house-keeping methods.

STREP THROAT: a contagious bacterial infection transmitted through sneezing, coughing, sharing of drinks, foods, utensils.

> Signs/Symptoms: sore throat pain with swallowing, fever, red swollen tonsils with white patches, small red spots on the roof of the mouth and swollen lymph nodes.
> Prevention: good personal hygiene, cover coughs and sneezes. Treatment includes antibiotics; do not return to school until fever free for 24 hours.

CONJUNCTIVITIS: "Pink Eye" can be a result of a virus, a bacterium, or an allergen. Viral conjunctivitis is highly contagious and spreads from hand to eye contact. Bacterial pink eye also can spread from person to person and is also spread by hand to eye contact by or contact with contaminated objects. Hay fever, asthma, and substances like contacts lens and its chemicals, cosmetics, and seasonal and environmental allergies are causes for allergens-based conjunctivitis. The distinguishing sign for bacterial conjunctivitis is a purulent (pus-like) discharge. Viral and allergen-based conjunctivitis produces clear watery discharge.

Signs/Symptoms: pink or redness to the white of the eye(s), increased tear productions, sensation of something in the eye, itching, burning, discharge, crusting of the eyes in the morning.

Prevention: wash your hands often, avoid touching your face with unwashed hands, as well as follow good hygiene health habits.

Blood Borne Pathogens (BBP)

Blood borne pathogens (BBP) are pathogenic microorganisms that are present in human blood and cause disease in humans through contact with infected blood or bodily fluids. The primary BBP diseases include Hepatitis B, Hepatitis C, and HIV. Bloodborne pathogens can enter the body through a break in the skin, sexual contact with infected person, sharing of razors or toothbrushes with infected person.

Universal Precautions include an approach to infection control to treat all human blood and certain human body fluids as if they were known to be infectious for HIV, HBV, and other bloodborne pathogens.

HBV: HEPATITIS B is a virus that effects the liver and is transmitted through contact with infected blood, or bodily fluids. HBV can survive outside the body at least 7 days and still be capable of causing infection. Symptoms begin an average of 90 days (range: 60–150 days) after exposure to HBV.

Signs/Symptoms: fever, fatigue, loss of appetite, nausea, vomiting, abdominal pain, dark urine, clay-colored bowel movements, joint pain, jaundice (yellowish skin and white of eyes)

Prevention: HBV vaccination (given at birth in U.S.)

HCV: HEPATITIS C is a blood-borne virus. Today, most people become infected with the Hepatitis C virus. Transmission can occur from sharing needles or other equipment to inject drugs, sexual partners, contaminated blood and blood products, body piercing, tattoos, and barbering.

Signs/Symptoms: fever, fatigue, loss of appetite, nausea, vomiting, abdominal pain, dark urine, clay-colored bowel movements, joint pain, jaundice (yellowish skin and white of eyes)

Prevention: No vaccine for hepatitis C is available.

HIV: HUMAN IMMUNODEFICIENCY VIRUS weakens a person's immune system by destroying important cells that fight disease and infection. In 2015, the CDC reported a slight increase in the number of cases of HIV. 80% of the cases were in the age group from 20-24. In 2017, the CDC reported the largest at-risk population for HIV is the college age student.

Signs/Symptoms: Flu-like symptoms include fever, chills, rash, night sweats, muscle aches, sore throat, fatigue, swollen lymph nodes, or mouth ulcers

Prevention: Abstinence is best method to prevent getting HIV from a sex partner. Practice safe sex. Follow universal precautions.

Fungal Pathogens

Fungal Pathogens are rarely dangerous, but some types can be harmful to your health. Mild fungal skin diseases typically present as a rash and are common in community-based environments.

"RINGWORM" is a common type of community based fungal skin infection. The shape of the circular ring-like rash gives the name "ringworm". The location of the fugal rash determines its name, such as "athlete's foot" is ringworm to the foot. Fungi pathogens thrive in dark moist environments. Transmission can occur from non-living objects to the skin. Fungal Infection can spread through shared towels, clothing, bedding, as well as hard surfaces, such as shower stalls, locker room floors, pool areas, etc. Secondary bacterial infections can occur from repetitive scratching of the itchy skin.

Signs/Symptoms: itchy, red, circular rash

Prevention: Basically, good personal hygiene habits along with good laundering and housekeeping methods is key.

"ATHLETE'S FOOT" is a fungal infection to the feet that often affects the space between the toes. Transmission sources are public showers, locker rooms, weight rooms, and wellness centers.

Signs/Symptoms: characterized by red and itchy skin fissures or scales.

Prevention: wear clean socks daily, dry feet after showering, avoid walking barefoot in public areas, locker rooms or public showers (wear sandals). Shower immediately after work outs, keep your workout clothes clean. Keep toenails clipped short and kept clean.

Parasitic Pathogens

Parasitic pathogens are organism that lives on or in a host and gets its food from or at the expense of its host. Some parasitic diseases are easily treated, and some are not.

BED BUGS are small, flat, parasitic insects that feed solely on the blood of people and animals while they sleep. Their slim flat bodies allow them to fit into the smallest of spaces and stay there for long periods of time, even without a blood meal. The bed bugs travel in the seams and folds of luggage, overnight bags, folded clothes, bedding, furniture, and anywhere else where they can hide. They hide during the day in places, such as seams of mattresses, box springs, bed frames, headboards, dresser tables, inside cracks or crevices, behind wallpaper, or any other clutter or objects around a bed. However, anyone who travels frequently and shares living and sleeping quarters where other people have previously slept has a higher risk of being bitten and or spreading a bed bug infestation.

Signs/Symptoms: The bite marks are similar to that of a mosquito or a flea -- a slightly swollen and red area that may itch and be irritating. The bite marks may be random or appear in a straight line. Other symptoms of bed bug bites include insomnia, anxiety, and skin problems that arise from profuse scratching of the bites.

Prevention: The best way to prevent bed bugs is regular inspection for the signs of an infestation. Practice good laundering and house-keeping methods.

SCABIES is an infestation of the skin by a human itch mite. The mite burrows into the upper layer of the skin where it lives and lays its eggs. The scabies mite usually is spread by direct, prolonged, skin-to-skin contact with a person who has scabies. Scabies sometimes is spread indirectly by sharing articles, such as clothing, towels, or bedding used by an infected person; however, such indirect spread can occur much more easily when there are crusted scabies.

Signs/Symptoms: intense itching, a pimple-like itchy rash, tiny blisters, and scales. Secondary skin infection from scratching the skin sores.

Sexually Transmitted Infections

Sexually transmitted infections (STI's) are transmitted through intimate sexual contact. Intimate sexual contact generally consists of vaginal sex, anal sex, and oral sex, although some diseases can be transmitted through hand/genital contact. Sexually transmitted infections are caused either by bacteria, viruses, parasites, or fungi. Bacteria, parasitic, and fungal STI's are curable while viral STI's are not curable, however they are treatable. STI's are most prevalent among people 15-24 years of age - most college students fall into this age range. Note, hormonal birth control methods DO NOT protect against STI's.

STI Risk Factors:

- ✓ Unprotected sexual intercourse (vaginal, anal, oral)
- ✓ Sharing of hypodermic needles
- ✓ Infidelity
- ✓ Many sexual partners (including serial monogamy)
- ✓ Alcohol/drug use prior to sex

Prevention:

- ✓ Abstinence
- ✓ Monogamy
- ✓ Regular use of latex condoms
- ✓ Open and honest communication between you and your partner
- ✓ Do not use alcohol or other drugs before or during sex
- ✓ Wash hands before sex
- ✓ Wash genitals after sex
- ✓ Urinate after sex

CHLAMYDIA

Signs/Symptoms: abnormal vaginal discharge; burning sensation when urinating; discharge from penis; pain and swelling in one or both testicles (although this is less common); and rectal pain, discharge or bleeding.

Pathogen: Bacteria

Transmission Mode: Fluid transfer; Vaginal; Anal; or Oral sex

Curable: Yes

Vaccine: No

GONORRHEA

Signs/Symptoms: burning sensation when urinating; white, yellow, or green discharge from the penis; painful or swollen testicles (although this is less common); increased vaginal discharge; vaginal bleeding between periods; anal discharge, itching, soreness, bleeding; and painful bowel movements.

Pathogen: Bacteria

Transmission Mode: Fluid transfer; Vaginal; Anal; or Oral sex

Curable: Yes

Vaccine: No

SYPHILIS

Signs/Symptoms: Primary: single or multiple sores: firm, round and painless that could last 3-6 weeks. Secondary: skin rash: looks red, reddish brown spots on the palms of your hands or bottom of your feet; rash will not itch but might be hard to notice; mucous membrane lesions. Tertiary: if left untreated, syphilis can cause damage to organs or organ systems include the cardiovascular system and central nervous system.

Pathogen: Bacteria

Transmission Mode: Skin-to-Skin Contact; Vaginal; Anal; or Oral sex

Curable: Yes

Vaccine: No

HPV

Signs/Symptoms: some cause genital warts; some cause cervical cancer and cancers to other parts of the body where the virus comes into contact

Pathogen: Virus

Transmission Mode: Skin-to-Skin Contact; Vaginal; Anal; or Oral sex

Curable: No, Genital warts can spontaneously disappear

Vaccine: Yes

HERPES

Signs/Symptoms: ***Oral (HSV-1):*** cold sores; sores/blisters in or around the mouth; may experience pain/itching at blister site; sores may crust over and form scabs; or sores/blisters may recur after a period of dormancy. ***Genital (HSV-2):*** sore/blisters in or around the penis, vagina, or anus; may experience pain/itching at blister site; sores may crust over and form scabs; sores/blisters may recur after a period of dormancy.

Pathogen: Virus

Transmission Mode: Skin-to-Skin Contact; Vaginal; Anal; or Oral sex

Curable: No

Vaccine: No

HIV

Signs/Symptoms: ***HIV: Early Stage:*** flu-like symptoms within 2-4 weeks of exposure; fever, chills, rash, night sweats; muscle aches; sore throat, swollen lymph nodes; fatigue; and mouth ulcers.

AIDS: rapid weight loss; recurring fever or profuse night sweats; extreme and unexplained tiredness; prolonged swelling of the lymph glands in the armpits, groin, or neck; diarrhea that lasts for more than a week; sores of the mouth, anus, or genitals; pneumonia; red, brown, pink, or purplish blotches on or under the skin or inside the mouth, nose, or eyelids; memory loss, depression, and other neurologic disorders.

Pathogen: Virus

Transmission Mode: Sharing Needles; Vaginal; Anal; or Oral sex

Curable: No

Vaccine: No

PUBIC LICE (CRABS)

Signs/Symptoms: itching in genital area; small, but visual bugs in your pubic area (including upper thighs); pubic lice eggs on the bottom part of pubic hair; dark or bluish spots on the skin where pubic lice are living; feeling of fever, fatigue, or irritable.

Pathogen: Virus

Transmission Mode: Skin-to-Skin Contact

Curable: Yes

Vaccine: No

Basics of First Aid CPR and AED Training

Basic first aid refers to the initial process of assessing and addressing the needs of someone who has been injured or becomes ill. Basic first aid allows you to quickly determine a person's physical condition and the correct course of treatment including activating the 911 system. Becoming first aid certified will help you identify when someone needs help and administer the correct care needed before medical professionals arrive. First aid certification will help you gain the skills required to help others during a wide range of emergencies. You will learn how to keep a person breathing, minimize consequences of injury or sudden illness and reduce their pain.

CPR and AED training will provide knowledge and skills necessary to save lives during an emergency situation. Performing CPR in the first few minutes of cardiac arrest can double or triple a person's chance of survival. According to the American Heart Association (AHA), "the average response time for first responders once 911 is called is 8-12 minutes. For each minute defibrillation is delayed, the chance of survival reduces by approximately 10%." Increasing public awareness of the importance of early intervention and ensuring greater public access to defibrillation will save many lives.

Cardiac Arrest

Cardiac arrest is an "ELECTRICAL" problem that causes the heart to malfunction and to unexpectedly stop beating. The electrical malfunction causes an irregular heartbeat which disrupts the heart's ability to pump blood to the brain, lungs and organs. Unresponsiveness occurs within seconds, breathing stops, and death occurs. If treated within a few minutes, cardiac arrest can be reversed in some victims.

Heart Attack

A heart attack is a "CIRCULATION" problem that occurs when blood flow to the heart is blocked. If the blocked artery is not reopened quickly, the part of the heart normally nourished by that artery dies due to lack of oxygen. Unlike with cardiac arrest, the heart usually does not stop beating during a heart attack. The longer the person goes without treatment, the greater the damage to the heart muscle. Symptoms can present gradually and persist for hours, days or weeks before a heart attack.

Signs and Symptoms of a heart attack include intense discomfort in the chest or other areas of the upper body, shortness of breath, cold sweats, and/or nausea/vomiting. Women symptoms may differ and include chest pain, shortness of breath, nausea/vomiting, and back or jaw pain.

The American Red Cross and the American Heart Association offer classes in CPR, AED, including Hands Only CPR.
Find a class at: **http://www.redcross.org/ux/take-a-class**

Chapter Summary

- ✓ Cardiovascular disease and cancer are the leading causes of death in the United States and their occurrence is related to heritable risk and various environmental stressors.
- ✓ Understanding how infectious diseases (viral and bacterial pathogens, blood borne pathogens, fungal and parasitic infections, sexually transmitted infections) are spread and taking the proper preventative steps significantly reduces risk.
- ✓ CPR and First Aid information can be found in various places and there are multiple avenues available for certification.

Chapter Review Questions

1) Define cardiovascular disease.
2) List risk factors for cardiovascular disease, and explain what lifestyle changes you can make to reduce your own personal risk.
3) Define cancer.
4) List risk factors for cancer and explain the choices you plan to make in order to limit your personal risk.
5) Describe the steps you can take to limit you risk of contracting and spreading community-based diseases.
6) What can someone who is not trained in CPR and first aid do in an emergency situation? Where can you go to receive that training and become certified?

References

About Cholesterol. (2017). Retrieved from **https://www.cdc.gov/cholesterol/about.htm**

About Heart Disease. (2017). Retrieved from **https://www.cdc.gov/heartdisease/about.htm**

About Stroke. (2017). Retrieved from **https://www.cdc.gov/stroke/about.htm**

American Stroke Association. (2017). Retrieved from **http://www.strokeassociation.org/STROKEORG/WarningSigns/Stroke-Warning-Signs-and-Symptoms_UCM_308528_SubHomePage.jsp**

Alcohol and Cancer Risk. (2013). Retrieved from **https://www.cancer.gov/about-cancer/causes-prevention/risk/alcohol/alcohol-fact-sheet**

Cancer-Causing Substances in the Environment. (2015). Retrieved from **https://www.cancer.gov/about-cancer/causes-prevention/risk/substances**

Cancer Prevention and Control. (2017). Retrieved from **https://www.cdc.gov/cancer/dcpc/prevention/index.htm**

Cancer Statistics. (2017). Retrieved from **https://www.cancer.gov/about-cancer/understanding/statistics**

Cold Sores: What You Need to Know. (2017). Retrieved from **https://www.webmd.com/skin-problems-and-treatments/ss/slideshow-cold-sores**

Common Cancer Types. (2017). Retrieved from **https://www.cancer.gov/types/common-cancers**

Coronary Angioplasty: Blockage in a Coronary Artery. (2010). Retrieved from **http://www.uofmhealth.org/node/650759**

Genital Herpes. (2017). Retrieved from **https://www.mayoclinic.org/diseases-conditions/genital-herpes/symptoms-causes/syc-20356161**

Healthy Eating for a Healthy Weight. (2016). Retrieved from **https://www.cdc.gov/healthyweight/healthy_eating/**

Heart Disease Fact Sheet. (2017). Retrieved from **https://www.cdc.gov/dhdsp/data_statistics/fact_sheets/fs_heart_disease.htm**

High Blood Cholesterol (2017). Retrieved from **https://www.nhlbi.nih.gov/health/resources/heart/heart-cholesterol-hbc-what-html**

High Blood Pressure. (2017). Retrieved from **https://www.cdc.gov/bloodpressure/index.htm**

HPV Infection. (2017). Retrieved from **https://www.mayoclinic.org/diseases-conditions/hpv-infection/symptoms-causes/syc-20351596**

Men and Heart Disease Fact Sheet. (2017). Retrieved from **https://www.cdc.gov/dhdsp/data_statistics/fact_sheets/fs_men_heart.htm**

Physical Activity for a Healthy Weight. (2015). Retrieved from **https://www.cdc.gov/healthyweight/physical_activity/**

Risk Factors for Cancer. (2015). Retrieved from **https://www.cancer.gov/about-cancer/causes-prevention/risk**

Sexually Transmitted Disease. (2017). Retrieved from **https://www.medicinenet.com/image-collection/crabs_pubic_lice_picture/picture.htm**

Sexually Transmitted Diseases. (2017). Retrieved from **https://www.cdc.gov/std/syphilis/default.htm**

STD (2017). Retrieved from **https://www.std-gov.org/stds/std.htm**

What are the Symptoms of Pubic Lice? (2017) Retrieved from **https://www.plannedparenthood.org/learn/stds-hiv-safer-sex/pubic-lice/what-are-symptoms-pubic-lice-crabs**

Skin Cancer Statistics & Fact. (2017). Retrieved from **http://www.skincancer.org/skin-cancer-information/skin-cancer-facts#men/women**

Types of Stroke (2017). Retrieved from **http://www.heartandstroke.ca/stroke/what-is-stroke**

Understanding Blood Pressure Readings (2017). Retrieved from **http://www.heart.org/HEARTORG/Conditions/HighBloodPressure/KnowYourNumbers/Understanding-Blood-Pressure-Readings_UCM_301764_Article.jsp#.WhHPjkqnGUk**

Warning Signs of a Heart Attack (2017). Retrieved from **http://www.heart.org/HEARTORG/Conditions/HeartAttack/WarningSignsofaHeartAttack/Warning-Signs-of-a-Heart-Attack_UCM_002039_Article.jsp#.WhHO0kqnGUk**

What is Cardiovascular Disease? (2017). Retrieved from **http://www.heart.org/HEARTORG/Support/What-is-Cardiovascular-Disease_UCM_301852_Article.jsp#.WhHLzUqnGUk**

What is Coronary Artery Disease? (2017). Retrieved from **https://www.nhlbi.nih.gov/health/health-topics/topics/cad/**

Chapter 10

Lifetime Physical Activity

By Tan Leng Goh, PhD and Amy G. Gagnon, EdD

Chapter Objectives

After reading this chapter, students should be able to:

- ✓ Understand what a Lifetime Physical Activity is;
- ✓ Know the various types of Lifetime Physical Activity; and
- ✓ Safely access a variety of Lifetime Physical Activities.

Maintaining a Lifetime of Physical Activity

"Movement is a medicine for creating change in a person's physical, emotional, and mental states."- Carol Welch

This chapter will discuss what Lifetime Physical Activity is and how it can positively affect an individual's physical, emotional, and social life. Many individuals prefer lifetime physical activity because these activities can be enjoyed by anyone regardless of age, athletic ability, or financial status. Another characteristic of lifetime physical activity is that both competitive athletes as well as those that perceive themselves as "non-athletes" may enjoy them.

Defining Lifetime Activities and its Importance

- ✓ PHYSICAL ACTIVITY - Physical activity is any body movement that works your muscles and requires more energy than resting. (NIH, 2016).
- ✓ PHYSICAL FITNESS - Good health and strength achieved through exercise. ("Recreation," n.d.)
- ✓ EXERCISE - Bodily or mental exertion, especially for the sake of training or improvement of health: ("Exercise," n.d.)
- ✓ LIFETIME PHYSICAL ACTIVITY - A variety of exercise/performance activities such that they will bring enjoyment and demonstrate the importance of maintaining health and wellness throughout the course of a lifetime.
- ✓ LIFETIME SPORTS_– a variety of sports that one can participate without physical contact or vigorous stress on the body.
- ✓ LEISURE/RECREATION - Time free from work or duties/ refreshment of strength and spirits after work. ("Recreation," n.d.)
- ✓ FLEXIBILITY- the ability to move a joint effectively through a range of motion (American Council on Exercise, 2018).

A primary goal of physically educating a student is to emphasize the importance of participating in physical activity for a lifetime. The college experience is the last opportunity faculty have to educate, promote, and provide a variety of activities in which students may select on their own, as a choice to lead a healthy life full of fun and movement. Engaging in any movement that allows our bodies to get stronger, be more flexible and perform daily living tasks with ease is vital to living a productive and healthy life.

There are countless benefits to exercising and engaging in physical activities including but not limited to: improving fitness levels, strengthening bones and muscles, stress reduction, and weight control (CDC, 2015). Lifetime physical activities are not different in this regard; however, the beauty of engaging in lifetime activities is that they do not require the individual to compete (unless chosen) and they do not require an organized team or specific facility in order to participate. Lifetime physical activities are exercises or activities that improve the physical, emotional and social state of a person that can be enjoyed at any age, young or old. Examples of lifetime physical activities and lifetime sports can be found below in Table 1.

Table 1. Examples of Lifetime Physical Activities

Hiking	Biking	Walking
Running	Geocaching	Weightlifting
Fitness training	Gardening	Swimming
Softball	Golf	Volleyball
Yoga	Rock climbing	Pickleball
Flag football	Ultimate Frisbee	Soccer
Basketball	Badminton	Tennis
Kite flying	Fishing	Bowling
Dancing	Archery	Martial Arts

As people age, their ability to compete in organized sport may end as the physical body loses strength, agility, balance, and quickness. Those skills are frequently used in organized, competitive sports. Although 480,000 college student-athletes compete in our country, the percentage going on to play professional sports is only between 0.9%-9.1% depending on the sport (NCAA, 2017). This number is drastically reduced when we look at those college students who do not compete on a team in college. The Centers for Disease Control and Prevention (2014) has estimated that only 1 in 5 adults meet the required 150 minutes of moderate intensity or 75 minutes of vigorous intensity of exercise per week and this number diminishes after graduation, emphasizing the need to find new interests after college in order to keep our bodies and minds strong and vibrant, as well as socialize.

Common myths about activity and aging (Robinson, Smith, & Segal, 2018) include:

(1) "There's no point to exercising. I'm going to get old anyway." In fact, maintaining a lifetime of physical activity can help an individual look and feel younger and stay independent longer;

(2) "Exercise puts me at risk of falling down." The truth is that lifetime physical activities help to build strength and stamina, prevent loss of bone mass and improve balance, thereby reducing an individual's risk of falling;

(3) "It's too frustrating: I'll never be the athlete I once was." Although strength and performance levels will decline with age, an individual can still derive a sense of achievement from lifetime physical activities for the improvement of health;

(4) "I'm too old to start exercising." Contrarily, adults who become active later in life often show greater physical and mental improvements than their younger counterparts.

As our adult responsibilities grow, the need for stress reduction becomes paramount and the opportunity to engage in activities that include competition and physical contact decline. Many people look to lifetime physical activities to remain physically and emotionally healthy, as well to seek out social opportunities. Lifetime physical activities can be as simple as taking a leisurely walk, gardening or practicing yoga. You are not limited to the activities we provided in Table 1. There are dozens of ways an individual may increase their physical activity levels during daily living tasks, such as parking further away to increase the number of steps to the store, taking the stairs instead of the elevator, and riding a bike instead of driving in the car.

It is important now to establish physically active habits. An individual's body will grow stronger from the time of birth until about the age of 30 (WebMD, 2018) where it then undergoes a decline in muscle mass. The decline of muscle mass is known as sarcopenia (0.5–1% loss per year after the age of 50). Sarcopenia is seen more so in individuals who lead an inactive lifestyle; however, it is evident in all individuals. Studies have revealed that physically inactive people can lose anywhere from 3-5% of their muscle mass each decade after their 30th birthday (WebMD). The primary treatment for sarcopenia is exercise, so be active now!

There are many physical and mental health benefits to maintaining a lifetime of physical activities. Physical benefits include helping individuals maintain or lose weight. Because metabolism slows with age, being physically active helps to increase metabolism, builds muscle mass, and burn more calories (see Table 2 below).

Table 2. Calories burned in various physical activities

	Calories used (burned) by a 154-pound man	
MODERATE physical activities:	In 1 hour	In 30 minutes
Hiking	370	185
Dancing	330	165
Weight training (general light workout)	220	110
Stretching	180	90
VIGOROUS physical activities:	In 1 hour	In 30 minutes
Bicycling (more than 10 mph)	590	295
Aerobics	480	240
Weight lifting (vigorous effort)	440	220

Source: www.choosemyplate.gov/physical-activity-calories-burn

Being physically active for a lifetime also reduces the impact of illness and chronic disease, such as improved immune and digestive functioning, better blood pressure and bone density, and a lower risk of Alzheimer's disease, osteoporosis, obesity, diabetes, heart disease, and certain cancers. Mental benefits include improved quality of sleep which is vital for an individual's overall health. Physical activities also helps to relieve stress, boosts mood and increases self-confidence. Engaging in regular physical activity as part of family life also provides children and parents with a strong foundation for a lifetime of health. Children who are physically active while they are young are likely to be physically active into their adulthood.

In addition to building muscle mass with physical activity, you can also improve flexibility and balance. As you learned in Chapter 2, flexibility is defined as the ability to move a joint effectively through a range of motion. The ability to bend, stretch, reach and move without limitation is necessary to not only exercise, but to successfully engage in daily tasks such as chores, carrying schoolwork to class, putting the dishes away and playing with children on the floor. Start engaging in daily stretching for even 10 minutes a day as a means to improve joint flexibility. Visit your app store for an easy to follow daily flexibility program such as Stretching and Flexibility Plan or 5 Minute Yoga Workouts.

Balance is defined by Merriam Webster as the even distribution of weight on each side of the vertical axis (2018). Balance is similar to stability, which you learned about in Chapter 2. Balance and flexibility can go hand in hand. Balance is imperative as it is necessary whether you are standing still or moving. Ones balance changes as we age and by gender. For females, balance tends to be easier as most females have shorter legs and wider hips providing a lower center of gravity and wider foundation on which to balance. As we age, balance becomes more important to avoid falls and continue moving safely especially when exercising. Exercises, sports and activities such as yoga, tai chi and simply engaging in physical activity every day will aid in the reinforcement of postural muscles used to balance every day.

Types of Lifetime Physical Activities

There are many different lifetime physical activities in which an individual may engage that can be competitive, non-competitive, free, or require little to no equipment. The choice is truly up to the individual and the benefits they hope to get out of the activity.

One avenue for engaging in physical activity is joining a fitness facility or local gym. Reasons for joining and paying for gym memberships may be to lose weight, maintain weight, or to reach specific athletic goals, such as training for a sport competition, obtaining a more appealing physique, or becoming stronger for daily functioning and working around the house. Whatever your goals are for visiting a fitness facility, keeping your body strong, flexible, and improving your cardiovascular system is paramount to living a healthy life. Please revisit the end of Chapter 2 for fitness facility descriptions and locations on campus which are free for students to use.

Other than joining a gym, there are alternative ways you can participate in weight training. In fact, weight training can include cardiovascular exercise (running on a treadmill, walking), resistance training (bands, bars), use of dumbbells and free weights or engaging in weight bearing fitness classes such as high intensity interval training (HIIT) or a combination of all the above. Recent statistics reveal that 80% of adults do not engage in any type of resistance training regimen (US Department of Health & Human Services). The *Journal of Medicine and Science in Sports and Exercise* (2011) found that individuals in their 60's and 70's were able to gain as much strength and muscle mass as those in their 40's, so it's never too late!

Yoga and any variation of a yoga class (yoga sculpt, core strength yoga, yoga fusion, etc.) appeal to many not only for the strength, flexibility, and postural benefits, but also equally as important, for the emotional benefits. Yoga provides participants with the ability to practice stress reduction, rest the mind of racing thoughts that occupy us each day, and an opportunity to breathe oxygen to all parts of our mind and body. Here at CCSU, please visit the RECentral website to learn about our Yoga and group fitness classes on campus: **www.ccsu.edu/recentral/FitnessClasses.html**

Martial arts such as judo, kickboxing, karate, taekwondo, jiu-jitsu, and krav maga are becoming popular in the United States. These activities can be learned by individuals through a trained instructor in facilities with the appropriate equipment. Lower impact martial arts such as tai chi and chi gong can be practiced by individuals into the later years of life because of its low impact on the joints, knees, neck, back, muscles and tendons.

Dance is another type of lifetime activity which can be enjoyed by many individuals. Different types of dance include ballet, barre, ballroom, and contemporary dance (jazz, hip hop, and world dance forms). Dance classes are available for children and adults.

Engagement in dance can help to increase muscular strength and endurance and motor fitness, aerobic fitness, muscle tone and strength, weight management, stronger bones and reduced risk of osteoporosis.

Walking or running is most commonly enjoyed by individuals who enjoy being outside and at a pace that is comfortable for themselves. Those that enjoy walking or running may use this form of lifetime physical activity as a means to also release stress and keep the body healthy. Some runners may enjoy a 5k run or even a half or full marathon. There is limited equipment needed provided the participant has a good pair of running shoes and the appropriate clothing for the season. Walking and running is great for the postural and core muscles, as well as the cardiovascular system!

Hiking, rock climbing, fishing, nature walks, and geocaching are most commonly enjoyed by nature enthusiasts! Being outside to enjoy the smells, sights, and sounds of nature provides a rejuvenation to the soul that being inside a fitness facility cannot mimic. Many are aware of what hiking and walking in nature is, but some may not be familiar with a newer activity called geocaching. Geocaching is a type of scavenger hunt using a global positioning system (GPS) device to find a target known as a cache. There are over 3 million geocaches hidden worldwide (3 million geocaches: the infographic, 2017). Using a smartphone application or handheld GPS, searchers may walk, climb or even swim to find the hidden cache. Many liken this activity to the new Internet game known as Pokemon Go, although it is different in many ways. For more information about geocaching, please visit **www.geocaching.org**.

Interested in more of a team or individual lifetime sport activity? Sports, such as tennis, bowling, swimming, volleyball, golf, pickleball and even ultimate Frisbee are widely played by adults at all ages! Depending on the sport, the equipment may vary and there could be a fee to enter a league or club in order to access the court, field or course. You can start becoming involved here at CCSU through participating in a Club sport or playing Intramurals; you can find information about both through the CCSU webpage.

Overall, the possibilities to continue moving, laughing, and enjoying time with others are bountiful. As your opportunities in college may soon come to an end, especially for student-athletes, consider learning a new physical activity or research where and how you can continue to enjoy your current activities. See activity #1 below to learn more about lifetime physical activities that might be possible for you now.

Activity #1:

Select three lifetime physical activities from Table 1: Examples of Lifetime Physical Activities and Sport. Then, define it, provide necessary equipment, cost, and ability to access in order to engage in the activity. A sample is provided for you below.

ACTIVITY	EQUIPMENT	COST	ABILITY TO ACCESS
SAMPLE: Hiking	Proper clothing, and hiking shoes/gear (if necessary)	None	Dependent on how near or far you are to a hiking trail.
Lifetime Physical Activity #1:			
Lifetime Physical Activity #2:			
Lifetime Physical Activity #3:			

Variety and Etiquette in Lifetime Physical Activities

Etiquette is practiced everywhere, not just at the dinner table. No one likes to share space with someone who may be loud, messy, or out of control with their body. Not only is this unsafe but it can also lead to injuries. Many people engage in physical activities to improve their mood and socialize with others. When someone enters their environment and does not follow established rules of that facility or is rude, it ruins the experience for many. Below is a list of general etiquette behaviors to follow when engaging in physical activity:

GENERAL ETIQUETTE BEHAVIORS:

- ✓ Keep your voice quiet or turned off unless you are with a partner who wants to talk with you.
- ✓ Wipe down exercise machines from any sweat or general germs you may have left behind.
- ✓ Do not wear street shoes inside a fitness or yoga facility. Cleanliness of exercise floors is important for safety, so leave those grass mowing sneakers at home!
- ✓ Respect everyone's personal space. If there are working machines open, select one not alongside another unless there are no other choices.
- ✓ Smile, be kind, and respect everyone's belongings. We are sharing space with others and we want to contribute to a positive experience for all.

Now you can go out there and visit a local fitness center, complete Activity #2 on your own to see what types of examples of etiquette you see out there.

Activity #2:

Visit a local fitness center (i.e. The "Y" or Big Sky or a CCSU facility) and provide three artifacts displaying etiquette, safety, and/or the fitness culture of the facility. Bring the three artifacts to show in class.

Safety in Physical Activity

When engaging in physical activity, environmental considerations, such as exercising in the heat, in the cold, in polluted air, and at high altitudes need to be taken into consideration and handled with care. As much as possible, avoid exercising outdoors in polluted air. Instead, exercising indoors on poor air quality days can avoid health problems such as increased risk of asthma development. If you engage in high-altitude physical activity, be sure to monitor onset of high-altitude sickness such as acute mountain sickness. To reduce the likelihood of high-altitude sickness, allow the body to slowly acclimatize to the altitude and keep hydrated.

When exercising in hot weather, your body undergoes a lot of stress. Both the exercise and the hot weather can increase your core body temperature to an unsafe level. As a result, heat-related illnesses (i.e., heat syncope-fainting, heat cramps, heat exhaustion, and heat stroke) can occur from exercising in extreme hot weather. Thygerson and Thygerson (2016) noted precautions to prevent heat-related illnesses:

- ✓ Exercise during the coolest times of the day
- ✓ Exercise in facilities with air conditioning
- ✓ Drink and replenish fluids lost from the body during exercise
- ✓ Wear lightweight and light-colored clothing
- ✓ Use sunscreen to protect against sun exposure
- ✓ Consider canceling or postponing exercise during extreme hot weather

When exercising in the cold, there is a risk of frostbite to your extremities (i.e., toes, fingers, nose, and ears) because blood is transferred toward the central organs to maintain core body temperature. Shivering is a sign of mild hypothermia. Thygerson and Thygerson (2016) noted precautions for exercising in the cold:

- ✓ Stay hydrated by drinking water; avoid alcohol and caffeinated drinks
- ✓ Wear multiple layers to keep warm and remove layers as necessary
- ✓ Wearing a hat can prevent heat loss from the head
- ✓ Socks, gloves, scarf, and face mask can be worn to protect extremities

Another safety precautions to note while exercising is overtraining. Signs of overtraining include general aches and pains that do not subside, muscle soreness, insomnia, inability to relax, dehydration, and falling sick easily. The first step to preventing overtraining is to slow down or stop exercising immediately. Remedies for muscle soreness include rest, ice, stretching, massage and heat application. If necessary, pain-relieving medications and topical creams can be purchased over the counter or prescribed by physicians to reduce muscle soreness.

If engaging in physical activity in a facility, be sure to read the rules and regulations pertaining to the safe use of the equipment so as not to result in injuries. In any exercise routine, be sure to wear the appropriate attire and footwear to engage in the exercise. Using inappropriate attire or footwear (for instance, shoes that are too uncomfortable for running) may result in injury (i.e., shin splint). Consult with professionals when purchasing attire, footwear, and equipment for the physical activity in which you are engaging.

Access to Physical Activities in Community, Campus, and at Home

When making decisions about engaging in physical activity at a fitness facility, consider the following steps (Thygerson & Thygerson, 2016): Costs of joining a fitness membership, cleanliness of the facility, availability of trained professionals with CPR certifications, length of time the facility has been in business (yes, some go out of business!), policies to withholding or ending memberships, distance from work or home, whether insurance reimbursement covers part or all of your membership, and whether the facility follows guidelines of the fitness industry.

Exercising in the comfort of our home is getting popular, especially with the increased use of Smartphone Applications and websites that promote physical activity. When choosing to exercise at home, considerations can be taken on the equipment needed. Some exercises that use body weight (i.e., yoga) involve low cost equipment, such as yoga/exercise mats, while others involve purchasing equipment that require adequate space at home. In purchasing equipment, considerations include buying machines or free weights/kettlebells/resistance bands. When buying exercise machines, there needs to be adequate space at home and they usually cost more than free weights. If cost is of concern, shop around for used fitness equipment through yard sales or consignment stores.

Activity #3:

Find 3 resources (i.e., websites and/or apps) that support regular leisure-time physical activity (i.e., Daily Yoga, Sworkit, etc.). Engage in the physical activity website/app and write a review about your experience using the website/app.

Barriers and Enhancers of Physical Activity

Attending college is a busy time of life but it is never too late to discover physical activities that we enjoy and want to engage for a lifetime! Nonetheless, there always exist obstacles in our lives that prevent us from leading a physically active lifestyle. Common barriers among college students are lack of time, lack of self-motivation, finding exercise boring, afraid of being injured, lack of self-management skills, and lack of accessibility to physical activity opportunities. Knowing the benefits of exercise far outweigh the barriers to exercising. Some strategies that can help you overcome the barriers may include:

- ✓ LACK OF TIME: Find "pockets" of time within your schedule to exercise. The Center for Disease Control suggest that a 10-minute bout of exercise at a time is fine.
- ✓ LACK OF MOTIVATION: Set goals, plan ahead, invite friends to exercise together, join a fitness class, reward yourself for achieving your goals.

- ✓ FEAR OF INJURY: Learn to warm up and cool down effectively to prevent injury, engage in a fitness class with a trained professional, and engage in low risk classes.

Now, it's your turn to list personal barriers and enhancers to engaging in physical activity (Activity #4)

Activity #4:

List some personal barriers and enhancers to engaging in physical activity. A sample is provided for you below.

NAME OF LIFETIME PA	BARRIERS TO PARTICIPATING	ENHANCER TO PARTICIPATING
SAMPLE: Geocaching	Might not have a smartphone	Get to be outside in nature and active
#1		
#2		
#3		

Chapter Summary

- ✓ Engaging in a variety of lifetime physical activities will bring enjoyment and maintain health and wellness throughout the course of a lifetime.
- ✓ A lifetime activity is a physical activity that can be enjoyed at all ages
- ✓ Individuals can choose different types of lifetime physical activities depending on their interest and environment.
- ✓ Etiquette, safety and access engaging in lifetime physical activity varies according to the chosen activity
- ✓ Identify various barriers and enhancers before engaging in lifetime physical activities.

Chapter Review Questions

1) How is a lifetime activity different from other physical activity?
2) List 3 different lifetime activities.
3) How can you keep yourself safe participating in the above 3 lifetime activities you listed?
4) List one barrier and one enhancer for each of the 3 lifetime activities you listed above.

References

American Council on Exercise (2018). What is Flexibility? Retrieved from **https://www.verywellfit.com/flexibility-definition-and-examples-3496108**

Centers for Disease Control and Prevention (CDC, 2014) Facts about Physical Activity. Retrieved from **https://www.cdc.gov/physicalactivity/data/facts.htm**

Centers for Disease Control and Prevention (CDC, 2015). Physical Activity and Health. Retrieved from **https://www.cdc.gov/physicalactivity/basics/pa-health/index.htm**

Exercise. (n.d.). Retrieved from **http://www.dictionary.com/browse/exercise**

Kettler, A. (2017, April 19). 3 million geocaches: The infographic. Retrieved from **https://www.geocaching.com/blog/2017/04/3-million-geocaches-the-infographic/**

Merriam Webster (2018) Retrieved from **https://www.merriam-webster.com/dictionary/balance**

National Collegiate Athletic Association (NCAA, 2017). Estimated probability of competing in professional athletics. Retrieved from **http://www.ncaa.org/about/resources/research/estimated-probability-competing-professional-athletics**

National Institutes of Health (NIH, 2016) What Is Physical Activity? Retrieved from **https://www.nhlbi.nih.gov/health/health-topics/topics/phys**

Recreation. (n.d.) Retrieved from **merriam-webster.com**

Robinson, L., Smith, & Segal, J. (2018). Senior exercise and fitness tips: No matter your age, it's never too late to get started. Retrieved from **https://www.helpguide.org/articles/healthy-living/exercise-and-fitness-as-you-age.htm**

Thygerson, A. L. & Thygerson, S. M. (2016). *Fit to be well: Essential concepts. 4th ed.* Burlington, MA: Jones and Bartlett Learning.

US Department of Health & Human Services. Retrieved from **https://www.hhs.gov/fitness/resource-center/facts-and-statistics/index.html**

WebMD (2018) Sarcopenia with Aging. Retrieved from **https://www.webmd.com/healthy-aging/guide/sarcopenia-with-aging#1**

Index